# TREATMENT PLANS AND INTERVENTIONS
# FOR OBSESSIVE-COMPULSIVE DISORDER

## TREATMENT PLANS AND INTERVENTIONS
## FOR EVIDENCE–BASED PSYCHOTHERAPY

Robert L. Leahy, Series Editor

*www.guilford.com/TPI*

Each volume in this practical series synthesizes current information on a particular disorder or clinical population; shows psychotherapists how to develop specific, tailored treatment plans; and describes interventions proven to reduce distress and alleviate symptoms. Step-by-step guidelines for planning and implementing treatment are illustrated with rich case examples. User-friendly features include reproducible self-report forms, handouts, and symptom checklists, all in a convenient large-size format. Specific strategies for handling treatment roadblocks are also detailed. Emphasizing a collaborative approach to treatment, books in this series enable therapists to offer their clients the very best in evidence-based practice.

TREATMENT PLANS AND INTERVENTIONS FOR DEPRESSION
AND ANXIETY DISORDERS, SECOND EDITION
*Robert L. Leahy, Stephen J. F. Holland, and Lata K. McGinn*

TREATMENT PLANS AND INTERVENTIONS FOR BULIMIA
AND BINGE-EATING DISORDER
*Rene D. Zweig and Robert L. Leahy*

TREATMENT PLANS AND INTERVENTIONS FOR INSOMNIA:
A CASE FORMULATION APPROACH
*Rachel Manber and Colleen E. Carney*

TREATMENT PLANS AND INTERVENTIONS
FOR OBSESSIVE–COMPULSIVE DISORDER
*Simon A. Rego*

# Treatment Plans and Interventions for Obsessive–Compulsive Disorder

Simon A. Rego

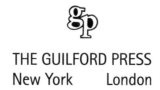

THE GUILFORD PRESS
New York      London

**Library of Congress Cataloging-in-Publication Data**

Names: Rego, Simon A., author.
Title: Treatment plans and interventions for obsessive–compulsive disorder / Simon A. Rego.
Description: New York, NY : The Guilford Press, [2016] | Series: Treatment plans
    and interventions for evidence-based psychotherapy | Includes bibliographical references
    and index.
Identifiers: LCCN 2016006009 | ISBN 9781462525683 (paperback : alk. paper)
Subjects: | MESH: Obsessive-Compulsive Disorder—therapy | Obsessive–Compulsive
    Disorder—prevention & control | Obsessive–Compulsive Disorder—diagnosis |
    Cognitive Therapy | Evidence-Based Medicine
Classification: LCC RC533 | NLM WM 176 | DDC 616.85/227—dc23
LC record available at *http://lccn.loc.gov/2016006009*

*For my incredible parents, Barbara and Tony*

*For my sister, Melanie, her husband, Jean,*
*and my beautiful niece, Scarlet*

*For my amazing Aunt Alice*

*And for the loves of my life, Adriana and Diego*

# About the Author

**Simon A. Rego, PsyD, ABPP,** is Director of Psychology Training and of the Cognitive Behavioral Therapy Training Program at Montefiore Medical Center, Bronx, New York, and Associate Professor of Clinical Psychiatry and Behavioral Sciences at Albert Einstein College of Medicine. Board certified in Cognitive and Behavioral Psychology by the American Board of Professional Psychology, he is a Fellow of the Academy of Cognitive Therapy and the Association for Behavioral and Cognitive Therapies, and a Founding Clinical Fellow of the Anxiety and Depression Association of America. Dr. Rego has authored numerous journal articles and book chapters on the treatment of obsessive–compulsive disorder and panic disorder and is a frequent presenter at national and international conferences.

# Preface

Most people reviewing a list of the common symptoms of obsessive–compulsive disorder (OCD) would likely be left wondering if they've been walking around undiagnosed for much of their lives. From experiencing an intrusive urge to act on some unwanted impulse to taking special measures to prevent or remove contact with contaminants, almost all of us will experience an occasional symptom of OCD. The difference between having this normal experience and having OCD is that people with OCD cannot dismiss these types of intrusive thoughts and cannot contain their need to perform rituals. So although the individual symptoms of OCD may seem harmless and even amusing to the general public, OCD can be so debilitating that the World Health Organization has ranked it among the 10 most disabling illnesses of any kind.

The good news is that we know more about OCD and its treatment now than at any other time in history. OCD has been studied in different age groups, across different races, ethnicities, and cultures, using different treatment approaches and formats. This work has led to a wealth of information on the nature of OCD and how best to treat it. For example, we now know that OCD is very common (the fourth most common psychiatric condition in the United States), with a lifetime prevalence of approximately 2.3%. And yet, we still struggle to get this information out to the patients who need it and to the mental health professionals who treat them. As a result, the bad news is that it takes an average of 14–17 years from the time OCD begins for people to obtain an appropriate diagnosis and treatment.

Fortunately, once a patient gets properly diagnosed, several promising psychological and pharmacological options are available for the treatment of OCD. In terms of psychological treatments, a behavioral approach called exposure and ritual prevention (Ex/RP) has been studied extensively around the world since the mid-1960s. Ex/RP is now considered to be the first-line psychological treatment for OCD—with more than four out of five patients being much or very much improved after finishing a full round of the treatment.

The premise behind Ex/RP is simple: have patients face the things (i.e., triggers, thoughts, and emotions) they have been avoiding, while at the same time preventing them from utilizing the rituals they have become used to employing to reduce their anxiety. This process allows *habituation* (a decrease in anxiety with the passage of time), and with it new learning, to occur.

Ex/RP has traditionally been carried out over the course of about 12–20 sessions. (Some researchers suggest that the amount of "homework" the patient does between sessions is a more important predictor of outcome than the number or duration of sessions.) In addition, the frequency of sessions (daily vs. weekly) and the format of the treatment (individual vs. group) do not appear to matter in terms of Ex/RP's effectiveness.

Patients who complete a full course of Ex/RP typically show rapid and significant improvement and then maintain the gains they made after the treatment. It seems to be equally effective for males and females of all ages and regardless of common demographic factors such as socioeconomic status or educational level.

Despite these impressive results, Ex/RP can be experienced as difficult and unpleasant work (i.e., a "bitter pill") for patients, with many studies reporting high dropout and refusal rates. Even patients who are much improved at the end of Ex/RP tend to have residual symptoms. On top of that, it can be difficult to find a mental health provider who is familiar with the treatment—and comfortable delivering it.

I wrote this book with these challenges in mind. I've been fortunate enough to work with some of the leaders in the field of OCD treatment over the years (e.g., Drs. Edna Foa, Jack Rachman, Arnold Lazarus, and William Sanderson) and, as a result, have experienced first-hand the powerful impact Ex/RP can have on the lives of patients suffering with OCD. However, I was also trained to do cognitive therapy for OCD and have seen the benefits of this approach as well. I have conducted OCD treatment in individual as well as group formats and have used different frequencies and durations for the treatment sessions. In recent years, I've also become a consumer of the research on "third-wave" treatment approaches (e.g., acceptance and commitment therapy, metacognitive therapy, mindfulness). As a result, I find myself not loyal to any particular theoretical approach. Rather, I try to understand the psychopathological mechanisms that the different theoretical approaches appear to be identifying and targeting, and then I wed the techniques and strategies from these approaches to maximize treatment outcome. I find that taking this approach also creates a certain freedom and flexibility in my clinical work.

In essence, this book is a reflection of my stance, written to serve as both a treatment manual and a treatment guide. My aim is to offer you a chance to learn how a typical course of Ex/RP can be structured, while also providing you with additional tools and resources that will allow you to adapt it to a specific patient's needs and to the context in which the treatment is going to be delivered. The book features a 16-session Ex/RP treatment protocol along with all the materials you need to carry out a course of treatment (e.g., reproducible assessment measures and patient handouts)—including strategies for overcoming motivational challenges and supplemental techniques and strategies taken from other evidence-based treatment approaches, including cognitive therapy, acceptance and commitment therapy, and metacognitive therapy. Having these additional techniques available should also help overcome many of the challenges I mentioned above and also create some flexibility in how the treatment is carried out. To illustrate how this balance can be achieved, I tie these various ideas together with a fictionalized case example that was created by combining symptoms from many of the patients I have treated in the past.

How, then, to start? While this book has been written for mental health practitioners across all fields and levels of training, it's important that you have at least some background familiarity with cognitive-behavioral therapy (CBT). Readers who are new to CBT may want to supplement their reading of this book with an introductory book on CBT (e.g., the excellent volumes by Ledley, Marx, & Heimberg, 2010, and Beck, 2011), sign up for few workshops on the principles of CBT, or find a supervisor familiar with the treatment for guidance. It's also important to remember that the session-by-session manual follows the chapters on assessment, diagnosis, clinical evaluation, and case formulation for a reason: to be truly competent and successful at treating OCD, you need to perform a thorough assessment and then generate a solid case conceptualization to serve as the blueprint for your treatment. Frequently, this conceptualization will suggest starting with Ex/RP. Occasionally, however, it will suggest starting with something else (e.g., motivational interviewing). Above all, you should be *personalistic* in your treatment—tailoring it to each individual patient by being willing to reassess and reconceptualize the case as you gain new information, and then being willing to adjust the treatment (e.g., weaving in additional techniques, switching to motivational interviewing, requesting a medication consultation) as necessary.

Patients with OCD desperately need access to more providers who understand how to implement the latest, evidence-based psychological treatments. I hope you enjoy reading this book and find that it helps create a sense that you're now a part of that group.

Please note: All case studies presented in this book are completely fictionalized amalgams of OCD cases I have treated over the past decade and a half. Any resemblance to real persons, living or dead, is purely coincidental.

# Contents

Purchasers of this book can download and print the forms in
Appendix B at *www.guilford.com/rego-forms* for personal use
or use with individual clients (see copyright page for details).

# List of Figures and Forms

## FIGURES

## FORMS

# CHAPTER 1

# Introduction
# to Obsessive–Compulsive Disorder

Obsessive–compulsive disorder (OCD) is a psychological disorder that is diagnosed based on the presence of either obsessions or compulsions (although, in most cases, both typically occur). Obsessions can take the form of thoughts (e.g., "That stain on the floor is dried blood!"), images (e.g., mutilated bodies), urges (e.g., to blurt out an obscenity in a formal setting), or impulses (e.g., to push an unsuspecting person in front a train). Note the repugnant, distasteful, and inappropriate nature of obsessions. They are typically much more bizarre and upsetting than everyday worries, and the individual usually knows that they don't make sense. Nevertheless, they occur over and over again and feel impossible to control and therefore become extremely anxiety-provoking and distressing. In an attempt to cope with these obsessions, the individual often tries to suppress or neutralize them in some way to make them go away—such as through use of repetitive behaviors or mental acts (i.e., compulsions or rituals) or through avoidance of situations that trigger the obsessions. Both obsessions and compulsions are time consuming and significantly interfere with the individual's ability to function in life.

OCD (by various names) has been noted in the literature for centuries. For example, persons with obsessive blasphemous or sexual thoughts were once considered to be *possessed*, as was consistent with the more religious worldview of the time and, as such, *exorcism* was considered the treatment of choice. Over the years, the explanation of obsessions and compulsions moved from a religious view to a medical view, which was formalized in 1838, when Jean-Étienne Dominique Esquirol (1772–1840) first described OCD in the psychiatric literature.

By the end of the 19th century, OCD was generally regarded as a manifestation of melancholy or depression, and by the beginning of the 20th century, theories of obsessive–compulsive neurosis shifted toward psychological explanations. In the first edition of the *Diagnostic and Statistical Manual of Mental Disorders* (DSM-I; American Pyschiatric Association, 1952), OCD was called "obsessive compulsive reaction." In DSM-II (American Pyschiatric Association, 1968), OCD was called "obsessive compulsive neurosis." With the publication of the DSM-III (American Pyschiatric Association, 1980), however, OCD as we now understand it was named and described. The definition only changed slightly in DSM-III-R (American Pyschiatric Association, 1987) and in DSM-IV (American Pyschiatric Association, 1994), and was not changed at all in the DSM-IV-TR (American Pyschiatric Association, 2000).

In DSM-5 (American Pyschiatric Association, 2013), however, OCD was removed from the anxiety disorders section and placed into a new, separate section called "obsessive–compulsive and related disorders." This section consolidated OCD with body dysmorphic disorder and trichotil-lomania, as well as newly added diagnoses of hoarding disorder and excoriation (skin-picking) disorder, and new diagnostic categories of substance/medication-induced OCD and OCD due to another medical condition. Also added was the following specifier, where indicated: With good or fair insight, with poor insight, or with absent insight/delusional beliefs. The decision to create a separate section for these disorders was based on the latest scientific evidence, which supported the interrelatedness of these disorders in terms of several diagnostic validators (e.g., symptoms, neurobiological substrates, familiality, course of illness, and treatment response) as well as the clinical utility of grouping these disorders in the same chapter.

Despite OCD being recognized in the medical literature over 175 years ago, historically, it has taken, on average, 14 to 17 years for people suffering with it to be accurately diagnosed and treated. This delay appears to be related to several factors, including (1) the tendency of many people to hide their symptoms, often in fear of embarrassment or stigma, and thus failure to seek seek help until many years after the onset of symptoms; and (2) the scant public awareness of OCD until recently, so that many people suffering from OCD were unaware that their symptoms were actu-ally part of a disorder that could be treated.

More recently, however, OCD seems to have caught the interest of the mainstream media, and, as a result, it has now been portrayed in characters in films (e.g., *The Aviator*, *As Good as It Gets*) and television shows (e.g., *Monk*, *Glee*); featured on documentaries and reality series (e.g., MTV's *True Life*, A&E's *Obsessed*, VH1's *The OCD Project*, A&E's *Hoarders*, and TLC's *Hoarding: Buried Alive*); and linked to a growing list of celebrities who have admitted having the diagnosis (e.g., Megan Fox, Alec Baldwin, Jennifer Love Hewitt, Howie Mandel, Howard Stern, Leonardo DiCaprio, Charlize Theron, Cameron Diaz, Billy Bob Thorton, and Jessica Alba). Although it is hoped that all of the media attention will ultimately be to the benefit of sufferers via an increase in awareness and destigmatization, it should be noted that some forms of OCD that are less "clas-sic" or common may not be so easily recognized by the public, the patient, the patient's family members, friends, or coworkers—or even seasoned therapists.

Complicating matters further is the research suggesting that the average person has approxi-mately 4,000 distinct thoughts in a typical waking day (16 hours), with approximately 500 of these thoughts being spontaneous, out of character, and experienced as intrusive (Klinger, 1978, 1996). In addition, this appears to be a global phenomenon: a recent study found that as many as 94% of people in 13 countries, across six continents, experience unwanted intrusive thoughts (Radomsky et al., 2014). There are also many people in community samples who report engaging in behaviors that could easily be classified as rituals, such as commuters who perform a check of their seat as they get up to leave a train or bus to "make sure" they did not leave something behind and people who use a public bathroom and place some form of barrier on the toilet seat or flush the toilet using one of their feet instead of one of their hands. Yet, not all of these people would be diagnosed with OCD.

Finally, in society today, we are constantly bombarded with stories in the press that con-tain warnings about the threats and dangers that are all around us, waiting to happen—all of which can encourage, if not create, compulsive-like behaviors. For example, we hear all the time about contamination hazards from bodily fluids and cleaning agents, dangers of radiation from cell phones, X-ray equipment, and computers, and the personal devastation caused by home invasions and robberies and, more recently, digital pickpocketing and identity theft. Constantly hearing this type of negative, sensationalized news can generate feelings of anxious apprehension, which in turn switches on our natural instinct to take action to make things safe. Yet, engaging in these types of behaviors would also not necessarily warrant a diagnosis of OCD.

*So what is OCD?* The above examples demonstrate an important fact of OCD (and most other mental health disorders): rather than being categorical in nature (i.e., either you have it or you don't), it is more dimensional (i.e., many of the defining symptoms are commonly found in most people, but it only crosses over into becoming a disorder at certain levels of severity). As such, it becomes important to understand the criteria used to determine when the symptoms of OCD move from being normal to being pathological.

## DIAGNOSTIC CRITERIA FOR OCD

To be diagnosed with OCD, an individual must experience *obsessions* or *compulsions* that are *severe enough* to cause a great deal of distress, interfere with the individual's life in some way (work, academic, social, etc.), and/or take up a lot of time (e.g., more than 1 hour a day). In addition, the *content* of the obsessions or compulsions cannot be better accounted for by another disorder (e.g., excessive checking to make sure the doors and windows are locked at night in a patient diagnosed with posttraumatic (PTSD) after being physically assaulted). Finally, the symptoms of OCD cannot be due to the direct effect of substance abuse, a medication, or a general medical condition. Please refer to the most recent version of the DSM for more detail on the diagnostic criteria.

## MOVING FROM NORMAL TO PATHOLOGICAL

As it is fairly common for people in societies around the world to experience unwanted intrusive thoughts and to engage in occasional rituals, establishing the presence of obsessions and/or compulsions is necessary but not sufficient to establish a diagnosis of OCD. The key step is to determine how much distress, disruption, or disability the experiencing of these symptoms is causing. To determine this effect, you can ask if the person is ever late in getting to work or school or in completing projects, papers, assignments, or tasks owing to obsessions or compulsions. In addition, you can also ask if the person's social life/relationships have been negatively impacted by the symptoms. Alternatively, you can ask the person to think of an average day and give an estimate of the total time he spends preoccupied with obsessive thoughts or engaged in compulsive behaviors. Finally, given that the person is presenting to you for help, you can typically assume he is experiencing a great deal of distress (unless his family, friends, or employer has pressured the patient into attending treatment).

## RULING OUT OTHER DIAGNOSES

Along with establishing the severity (i.e., distress, disruption, or disability) of the symptoms, it's important to remember that a diagnosis of OCD should not be given if the content of the obsessions or compulsions is better accounted for by another psychological disorder. For example, symptoms resembling OCD that would not warrant a diagnosis of OCD include repetitive hair pulling in a patient diagnosed with trichotillomania; obsessive thoughts about having a disease or illness along with excessive medical check-ups in a patient diagnosed with either somatic symptom disorder or illness anxiety disorder; or obsessive thoughts about food in a patient diagnosed with an eating disorder. In addition, the symptoms of OCD must not be due to the direct effect of substance abuse (e.g., cocaine), a medication (e.g., thyroid medications), or a general medical condition (e.g., Parkinson's disease, brain injury).

In some cases, however, symptoms that mimic OCD that are better explained by another disorder may appear *in addition to* other symptoms of OCD that are *not* better explained by this disorder. As a result, it is important to be knowledgeable of common comorbid conditions and thorough and detailed in your assessment in order to make a precise differential diagnosis. This issue will be discussed in more detail in Chapters 2 and 4.

## SPECIFIERS

Individuals with OCD differ in their level of understanding about the accuracy of the thoughts, images, impulses, or urges central to their disorder. The DSM refers to these different levels of understanding as different levels of *insight*, which can range from good to absent. In brief, the poorer the insight (i.e., the less a patient recognizes his or her obsessions as unreasonable), the greater the chance that treatment of the patient will be challenging. Please refer to the most recent version of the DSM for more detail on the different specifiers that can be used to account for differing levels of insight.

Also, insight can vary *within a patient* over the course of the illness (again, with poorer insight generally being linked to worse treatment outcome). Thus, at certain times an individual patient may acknowledge that his symptoms are unreasonable and/or excessive, whereas at other times that same patient may be totally convinced that his beliefs are true! Thus, throughout the treatment it is important to check in from time to time on the patient's level of understanding about the accuracy of his obsessions.

Finally, when the individual has a history of a *tic disorder*, you should use the specifier "tic-related" (the DSM notes that up to 30% of individuals with OCD have a lifetime tic disorder and that this condition is most common in males with onset of OCD in childhood).

## RATIONALE FOR COGNITIVE–BEHAVIORAL TREATMENT

As will be discussed in more detail in Chapter 2, the exact cause of OCD remains unknown. Perhaps that is why many competing theories have emerged over the years, often espousing very different approaches to treatment. This competition likely helped fuel the significant advances that have been made in the treatment of OCD. In just the past 30–40 years, for example, our notion of OCD has moved from that of a disorder that came with a poor prognosis to one in which many patients can expect to see a significant response to treatment and, occasionally, a total remission of the disorder). At the same time, it has also made it confusing for patients (and clinicians) to know which approach to begin with when starting treatment of OCD.

Fortunately, various expert consensus guidelines have been written over the years to aid in the treatment selection for patients diagnosed with OCD (e.g., March et al., 1997; National Institute for Health and Clinical Excellence, 2005; Nathan & Gorman, 2015; *www.psychologicaltreatments.org*). Of the many different psychological treatments offered for OCD, cognitive-behavioral therapy (CBT) in general, and exposure and ritual prevention (Ex/RP) in particular, have the strongest evidence base. As such, a consistent recommendation found in the expert consensus guidelines is to start treatment with CBT alone or in combination with a medication, with the likelihood that a medication will be included in the recommendation varying as a function of both the severity of the OCD and the age of the patient. For example, for milder forms of OCD, starting treatment with CBT alone appears to be the expert consensus. As the severity of the OCD increases, however, expert consensus guidelines are more likely to suggest adding a medication to CBT as the initial treatment—or even starting with medication alone. Similarly, for younger patients, as the patient's age decreases, expert consensus guidelines are more likely to suggest using CBT alone.

CBT, with its focus on cognitions (e.g., obsessions, mental rituals) and actions (e.g., behavioral rituals) and their connection to emotions (e.g., anxiety), lines up nicely with the DSM criteria for OCD. In addition, CBT's emphasis on the present, providing patients with education about their disorder, and being more actively involved as a therapist can be utilized to "meet patients where they are," normalize their symptoms, and encourage patients to become active collaborators in their treatment. Together, these elements serve to instill hope and increase motivation for change—even in patients who have suffered with the disorder for years.

CBT is, however, a challenging treatment for some patients to embrace. In fact, critics of CBT point out that some studies using Ex/RP for OCD have very high patient dropout rates. As such, it is very important for clinicians who are new to this treatment to understand how it works, so that they may first present it to their patients in a way that demonstrates an understanding of, and confidence in, both the CBT model and treatment components and then be able to anticipate any potential problems, concerns, or issues that their patients may experience. If the treatment is presented properly, patients hearing it will likely feel anxious about the short-term challenges that lie ahead, but confident in the therapist's ability to help them get through it, as well as their long-term prognosis.

## USING THIS TREATMENT PLANNER

This book is intended to be a comprehensive guide for clinicians who wish to take an evidence-based approach to the treatment of OCD. Experienced clinicians, new professionals, and graduate students should all find useful information within this planner to guide their treatment of OCD. Although no prior training in CBT is required for use of this treatment planner, a basic knowledge of the key concepts of CBT will be useful for any practitioner. Interested readers should refer to Appendix A (Resources) for suggested readings.

Included in this treatment planner are the diagnostic criteria for OCD; background information on the conceptualization and treatment of OCD; assessment tools; patient handouts and worksheets; a session-by-session treatment manual for clinicians wanting to know the "nuts and bolts" of conducting Ex/RP; a chapter containing supplementary techniques from cognitive therapy, acceptance and commitment therapy, and metacognitive therapy; and an extensive case example to illustrate the treatment plan in action. Used together, these materials will equip you to assess, diagnose, conceptualize, and treat a patient with OCD, using Ex/RP as a backbone and supplementing with additional techniques when necessary.

Before providing this treatment, you should be familiar with the entire treatment protocol. In addition, consistent with ethical guidelines for clinical conduct, you should seek clinical supervision prior to treating an individual when the presenting problems are outside the bounds of your expertise.

Despite the rise of alternative psychological treatments, it is important to note that Ex/RP remains the "treatment of choice" for OCD. As such, it is strongly recommended that you use the cognitive-behavioral treatment plan described in detail in this planner first, in conjunction with a detailed assessment and case formulation (see Chapter 4), for the appropriate target population (adults and adolescents with a primary diagnosis of OCD, in an outpatient treatment setting).

Of course, it is expected that you will adapt the treatment to fit each patient's unique symptoms and needs, and will augment the treatment with additional evidence-based treatment components as roadblocks are encountered. To support your individualizing each client's care, I make suggestions for incorporating components from other evidence-based treatments into the treatment. Thus, the included treatment planning materials represent a synthesis of Ex/RP, the gold-standard treatment for OCD, along with more recent innovations that have burgeoning empirical bases.

In this introductory chapter, I have discussed the history of OCD, explored the diagnostic criteria of OCD, defined obsessions and compulsions, and provided basic information about CBT and its application to OCD. In Chapter 2, I expand on the essential features and give examples of subtypes of OCD, discuss comorbid conditions and differential diagnosis, provide a review of the epidemiology of OCD, and summarize several different theories that have been offered to explain the etiology and maintenance of OCD.

Chapter 3 reviews the various evidence-based treatments for OCD, including biological treatments (e.g., pharmacotherapy, stereotactic neurological procedures, subconvulsive stimulation treatments) and psychological treatments (cognitive therapy, behavioral therapy, with and without various medications) in different formats of delivery and treatment settings.

Chapters 4 and 5 present a detailed discussion of how to use diagnostic and clinical evaluations to aid in the assessment, diagnosis, and case formulation and, in so doing, maximize the potential for a positive treatment outcome.

Chapter 6 provides a detailed overview of the treatment plan, with Chapters 7–13 presenting session-by-session suggestions for implementing Ex/RP for OCD, including thorough descriptions of interventions, in-session worksheets, patient handouts, and suggestions for between-session homework. Although this 16-session treatment manual has been written for adult and adolescent patients seeking outpatient treatment for OCD, it can also readily be adapted for younger or older patients.

Chapter 14 includes a summary of additional techniques taken from three other evidence-based treatments (cognitive therapy, acceptance and commitment therapy, and metacognitive therapy) that can be used to supplement the core treatment.

Chapter 15 offers a case example that parallels the session-by-session treatment planner.

Chapter 16 offers a summary, some reminders and concluding remarks, and of course, a few final take-home messages!

Finally, in the two appendices you will find resources (readings, websites, sources for expert consensus guidelines, and lists of empirically based self-report measures) and reproducibles (forms and handouts) that will help you in the delivery of the treatment.

---

## TAKE-HOME MESSAGE

If we start to view OCD "symptoms" as global and universal phenomena, we can learn a few valuable lessons about the assessment, diagnosis, and treatment of patients with OCD. First, we must keep in mind that intrusive thoughts and compulsions are *common*—almost all people experience occasional symptoms that are, in content, no different from those of patients diagnosed with OCD. As a result, OCD is a disorder that is best viewed in a *dimensional* rather than *categorical* manner. Second, in order to move from normal to abnormal, the symptoms of OCD must take up a significant amount of time, cause significant distress, or significantly impact on the person's work functioning, social life, or home responsibilities. Third, many other psychological, medical, and substance-related disorders can generate symptoms that resemble those found in OCD. As such, a careful screening should be conducted to allow for a meaningful differential diagnosis and consideration of comorbid disorders. Lastly, patients' insight into the nature of their OCD is often dynamic. As a result, it may be useful to view the patient's level of insight about her symptoms as fluctuating on a spectrum, ranging from seeing them as normal intrusive thoughts to believing 100% that they are true (i.e., delusional thinking). It may also prove useful to inquire about whether a patient's insight has shifted over the course of the disorder. Of the many different psychological treatments offered for OCD, CBT, in general, and Ex/RP, in particular, have the strongest evidence base and, as such, treatment should begin with Ex/RP—either alone or in combination with a medication.

---

# CHAPTER 2

# Understanding
# Obsessive–Compulsive Disorder

Recall from Chapter 1 that OCD consists of recurring obsessions, compulsions, or both. The obsessions in OCD are recurrent thoughts, images, urges, or impulses that a person experiences as unwanted, distasteful, inappropriate, intrusive, and distressing, whereas the compulsions in OCD are behaviors or mental acts that the person feels driven to perform repeatedly and rigidly in an attempt to "neutralize" an obsessive thought by either preventing the feared consequence or relieving the anxiety caused by it. Over the years, researchers have grouped the symptoms reported by patients into several categories as a way of facilitating assessment and treatment. These categories are described in detail below, followed by the epidemiology, prevalence, and life course of OCD, theories of OCD, and finally, understanding OCD in cognitive-behavioral terms.

Obsessions can be grouped into several categories:

1. *Fear of contamination.* This is the most frequently reported category of obsessions, with the most common examples being an excessive concern with dirt or germs—either in general or from something more specific (e.g., asbestos, household cleaners and solvents, computer radiation). This category can also include less common examples, such as being excessively concerned with impregnating another person.

2. *Doubting one's actions or conversations.* This is the second most frequently reported category of obsessions, with the most common examples being an excessive concern about whether a door was left unlocked, an appliance was left plugged in, or a faucet was left running. This category can also include almost any routine activity after which the person wonders whether she wasn't careful enough, performed it correctly, or, at times, even did it at all—and then typically fears that this in turn could cause something awful or harmful to happen to others, such as an accident or injury.

3. *Unacceptable thoughts or impulses directed toward oneself or others.* This category contains themes of aggressive, violent, or sexual thoughts or impulses, as well as ideas of religious blasphemy and/or sacrilege. Before providing examples, it is important to note that many therapists unfamiliar with this category of obsessions react to disclosures of these types of thoughts by immediately conducting assessments of the patient's safety or dangerousness. Unfortunately, in patients with

OCD, this type of reaction can inadvertently strengthen their conviction that they really could be a danger to themselves or to others. Recall that, by definition, obsessions are experienced as unwanted, intrusive, and distressing. These components should be kept in mind when individuals reporting these types of thoughts are screened, as they can help differentiate OCD-related thoughts from thoughts commonly associated with other mental health disorders (e.g., a patient with conduct disorder or antisocial personality disorder will not likely experience violent thoughts as intrusive or upsetting). As a result, careful questioning related to the nature of the thoughts, balanced with psychoeducation, normalizing, and a rationale for asking about them in patients with OCD, is called for in these cases.

Common examples of aggressive or violent thoughts in patients with OCD include doing something to harm a loved one (e.g., drowning a child), a vulnerable person (e.g., pushing an unsuspecting elderly person in front of a train), or oneself (e.g., swerving a car off the road while driving, hanging oneself), but can also include other disturbing images (e.g., sexual assault, mutilated bodies in car crashes). Common examples of sexual obsessions include engaging in a sexual act that is personally disgusting (e.g., incest) and experiencing urges to engage in unsolicited sexual acts with others (e.g., touch a stranger's genitals, buttocks, or other "private" parts, make a sexually crude comment to a stranger). Examples can also include doubts about one's sexuality (e.g., whether one is a child molester) or sexual orientation (e.g., heterosexuals with homosexual images or urges, homosexuals with heterosexual images or urges). When assessing for sexual obsessions, it is important once again to note that obsessions are experienced as unwanted and intrusive and therefore should be distinguished from sexual fantasies which, though not always falling into "traditional" or widely expressed ideas about sex, are nevertheless pleasurable and therefore not experienced as intrusive.

Finally, common examples of religious obsessions include engaging in a sacrilegious act (e.g., violating a sacred object), experiencing unwanted blasphemous impulses (e.g., cursing God, yelling out something during a religious ceremony or while praying), having ideas of being condemned to Hell, and feeling doubts in adequately following religious principles. When assessing for religious obsessions, it can often be useful to consult with a religious leader in the patient's community, especially when working with people with religious views differing from your own.

4. *Concerns about symmetry, ordering, completeness, exactness, the need for things to be "just right," and the need to maintain a rigid routine.* The most common examples of this category include experiencing an excessive concern about one's belongings not being touched or moved, needing things to be organized in a particular way (e.g., being bothered if pictures are not straight or books are not lined up on a bookshelf), and speaking or writing words in a specific way in order to get them "just right." This category can also include making sure that one is dressed or groomed in a perfectly symmetrical manner, seeing that objects are placed on surfaces in specific ways, and/or maintaining highly specific and rigid exercise, eating, or bathroom routines.

5. *Other, "miscellaneous" obsessions that don't fit neatly into one of the above categories.* The most common examples include having lucky or unlucky numbers (e.g., 7 is lucky and 13 is unlucky), needing to know or remember trivial/nonessential details (e.g., house numbers, license plates), attributing special significance to certain colors (e.g., black = death, red = blood), and harboring superstitious fears (e.g., stepping on sidewalk cracks, spilling salt). This category can also include

any other thoughts (e.g., phrases from a movie), images (cartoon characters' faces), or sounds, words or music (e.g., a song with no significance) that contain the components of an obsession.

Finally, it should be noted that the term *obsession* has also found its way into today's vernacular. In this context, however, the term is often used to convey a strong interest in something (or someone) to the point that all else fades in significance. The important distinction is that in these cases the interest is typically not experienced as unwanted, intrusive, or repugnant and often generates feelings of excitement and pleasure rather than anxiety and distress. As a result, the person does not typically make any effort to resist or dismiss it.

As with obsessions, compulsions can also be grouped into several categories:

1. *Frequent washing and cleaning.* This is one of the top two most frequently reported categories of compulsions. The most common examples in this category are excessive or lengthy hand washing or showering, and house cleaning. This category can also include taking special measures to prevent contact with dirt or other perceived contaminants or pollutants (e.g., wearing gloves, opening a bathroom door using a paper towel in the hand, using a foot to flush a public toilet, not sitting near "contaminated" people on buses or trains or in waiting areas) or following rigid routines (e.g., cleaning body parts in a certain order in the shower, wiping a specific way after using the toilet, or removing clothes in a set pattern when getting undressed after work/being outside of the home) in order to prevent spreading contamination.

2. *Checking more than is necessary.* This is the other of the top two most frequently reported categories of compulsions. The most common examples in this category include checking to ensure the safety of one's physical surroundings (e.g., doors being locked, windows being closed, appliances being unplugged, stove being turned off), as well as checking that one did not inadvertently harm others (e.g., looking in the rear view mirror of the car to make sure a pedestrian was not hit without the person realizing it). This category can also include checking to make sure that one did not intentionally or accidentally harm oneself (e.g., stabbed self with a knife, overdosed on medications); did not make a mistake (e.g., reviewing e-mails or written assignments); and did not inadvertently do or say something to insult someone (e.g., mentally reviewing past events or conversations).

3. *Repeating specific phrases or redoing certain routine actions.* The most common examples in this category include turning light switches on and off, sitting down and getting up in chairs, and walking in and out of doorways. This category can also include almost any routine action (e.g., placing objects down on a table, repeating words, phrases or prayers either mentally or out loud) that is repeated until it feels "just right."

4. *Counting compulsions.* The most common example involves having strong preferences for certain numbers. This category can also include rituals such as counting senseless things such as the number of ceiling tiles or the number of people in a room, the number of letters in each word while reading, or the number of steps one takes between two destinations (e.g., the subway stop and the front door of the office).

5. *Arranging and ordering things such that they are straight, sequenced, or in a certain order.* The most common examples include having cans lined up in a cabinet, arranging towels by color, and

making sure hanger hooks all face a certain direction. This category can also include eating foods in a particular order and making sure all of one's picture frames are perfectly straight and books are organized (by category, author, title).

6. *Needing to ask, tell, or confess.* The most common examples of this category include repetitively seeking reassurance from—or for the opinion of—others (e.g., about a health-related concern or the safety of engaging in a given activity). This category can also include needing to tell or confess one's perceived wrongful acts or thoughts (e.g., confessing to a crime one did not commit, confessing minor religious infractions to a holy leader, being "compulsively" honest with a loved one) or asking a seemingly endless number of questions until the other person (e.g., teacher, friend, stranger) becomes annoyed or irritated.

As I noted earlier when discussing the term "obsession," the term "compulsive" has also found its way into today's vernacular. In this context, however, the term is often used to convey the idea that the person in question has difficulties resisting impulses to lie, gamble, steal, and so on, or performing various body-focused repetitive behaviors such as hair pulling, skin picking, and nail biting. In the case of impulses, the behaviors tend to lack the characteristic features of OCD-type compulsions, such as resistance of the urge, reluctance to carry out the behavior, and not deriving any pleasure from the act. In the case of body-focused repetitive behaviors, the behaviors tend to lack the characteristic features of OCD-type compulsions, as they often occur without awareness or in the context of affect dysregulation.

Finally, as I described in Chapter 1, based on the diagnostic criteria, a patient does not need to have both obsessions and compulsions in order to be diagnosed with OCD. Although the majority of patients presenting for treatment report experiencing obsessions and engaging in compulsions, there do appear to be a smaller but significant percentage of patients who seemingly do not fit this model. These patients can be categorized into three groups: (1) "pure obsessionals," (2) those who engage only in mental compulsions, and (3) patients with "primary obsessional slowness."

## PURE OBSESSIONALS

These patients report experiencing a form of OCD characterized primarily by repetitive intrusive thoughts. Some researchers have described them as "pure obsessionals," to reflect the idea that they only report experiencing obsessions (e.g., "Am I really alive?" or "I could stop breathing at any moment!") but deny engaging in any form of compulsion in response to the obsessions. This is a somewhat controversial category, with some researchers believing these individuals in fact do engage in compulsions, but that these compulsions are mental and thus covert, which makes them very difficult to observe.

## PATIENTS WHO ENGAGE ONLY IN MENTAL COMPULSIONS

Although many people think of obsessions as mental phenomena and compulsions as overt behavioral acts, there are in fact a sizeable proportion of patients whose OCD is characterized primarily by mental compulsions, with few if any overt behavioral rituals. One group of these patients engages in covert, mental compulsions to seek relief from their obsessions (e.g., reciting a prayer silently to themselves, repeating a "good" thought in order to counteract a "bad" or immoral thought, or reviewing prior conversations to make sure they didn't offend anyone). However, another group of these patients appears to engage in covert, mental compulsions that are not triggered by any clearly identifiable obsessions.

## PATIENTS WITH PRIMARY OBSESSIONAL SLOWNESS

According to some researchers, there are a small number of patients whose key symptom involves "primary obsessional slowness." They suffer from a type of OCD in which their slowness is the primary problem rather than those problems arising from engaging in the compulsions of OCD. These patients were first described around the mid-1970s and tend to be male. They typically engage in extremely meticulous and precise behaviors, primarily involving self-care and other simple daily tasks (e.g., brushing teeth, bathing, dressing, grooming), with each task having to be performed in a specific and rigid, self-prescribed manner.

## EPIDEMIOLOGY, PREVALENCE, AND LIFE COURSE OF OCD

Data on the prevalence of OCD suggests that 2.3% of Americans will be diagnosed with OCD at some point in their adult lives. In addition, studies examining the impact of culture on OCD in the United States have not found any differences in prevalence of OCD based on race (Hispanic, African American, white), although epidemiological data have indicated that OCD is slightly less common among African Americans than whites in the general population. This difference does not appear to be significant, however. As a result, some researchers suggest that differences in the observed prevalence rates of OCD between cultural groups in the United States may be due to greater tolerance in some cultures for behavior that deviates from the norm.

Lifetime prevalence rates of OCD are also remarkably consistent for other cultures around the world, such as Puerto Rico, Canada, Germany, New Zealand, and Korea. The exception is Taiwan where the rates are substantially lower, but this may be due to methodological differences in the epidemiological studies. Women appear to develop OCD slightly more frequently than men (e.g., they have a lifetime prevalence of 2.9% vs. 2% in men), whereas among children, boys tend to have a higher prevalence rate than girls.

OCD tends to start in adolescence, with the majority of patients experiencing the onset of symptoms before age 25. Although the symptoms tend to develop gradually, an abrupt onset of OCD has sometimes been observed in postpartum mothers. If left untreated, the course is typically chronic, with some fluctuation in the severity of symptoms over time. For example, in one study of 560 patients, it was found that 85% of the OCD patients had a continuous course with waxing and waning symptoms and 10% had a deteriorative course, while only 2% had an episodic course marked by full remissions lasting 6 months or more (Rasmussen & Eisen, 1992).

Given its relatively high prevalence (the fourth most common psychological disorder) and chronic course if left untreated, it may come as no surprise that the World Health Organization lists OCD as one of the top 10 disabling conditions in the world. What may come as a surprise, however, is that this list includes physical ailments—a fact that highlights the devastating global impact that OCD can have on one's life. One study, published in 1995, estimated the total costs of OCD at $8.4 billion in 1990, with indirect costs (e.g., lost productivity) estimated at $6.2 billion.

# THEORIES OF OCD

Mr. Smith has struggled with symptoms of OCD for years. He recalls, even as a young child, needing to touch something white immediately after touching anything black and needing to turn the light switch in his bedroom off and on seven times before going to bed—or else he would get very stressed out and end up having a tantrum. Although these symptoms resolved over the years, as he entered into adulthood, new symptoms seemed to emerge, including the need to check the door locks and windows several times before leaving his home and before going to bed, and to only read books he owned with gloves on. He knows there is no rational reason for these behaviors, but nonetheless feels compelled to carry them out and is unable to resist performing them.

What is it about Mr. Smith that differentiates him from someone else who does not suffer from OCD? Is it something in his genetic makeup? Is his brain wired differently? Is it the way he was raised? What factors play a role in the etiology and perpetuation of OCD? The following sections will look at some of the factors thought to make individuals more or less vulnerable to developing OCD and then explain how OCD symptoms, once triggered, can be maintained over time.

## Genetic Factors

It's tempting to attribute all differences between one person and another to genes. Recent advances in technology have given us a clearer glimpse into what genes are, how they function, and the kind of impact they have on the development of our minds and bodies—not to mention on our behavior. What do genetic studies tell us about OCD? Is this a disorder that's handed down from one generation to another?

One way in which researchers have attempted to determine whether genetic factors play a role in the development of OCD is by examining data from twin studies. Researchers typically compare the rate at which disorders appear in monozygotic ("identical") twins and in dizygotic ("fraternal") twins. In the case of OCD, the data from some twin studies suggest a higher rate of concordance for monozygotic twins, although there are contrasting findings. In addition, some researchers have examined the rate of OCD among immediate (i.e., first-degree) relatives and found that it is considerably higher (about 25%) than would be expected by chance, whereas other researchers have found a higher rate of psychiatric disorders in general—including anxiety disorders—but not necessarily higher rates of OCD per se.

Therefore, although there is evidence that genes play a role in the development of psychiatric disorders in general, many experts suggest that the genetic contribution may be better explained as creating a general tendency to behave fearfully (i.e., "anxiety sensitivity"), which can predispose an individual to developing some form of anxiety disorder. Experts also suggest that some other factor in the environment (e.g., learning) may then determine the specific form of the anxiety disorder as well as the particular ways in which the individual will attempt to manage it. For an excellent review, along with the results of the first genomewide association study (GWAS) of OCD, see the work of S. Evelyn Stewart et al. (2013).

## Biological Factors

Although the evidence suggests that individuals with OCD differ from those without OCD in a number of biological features, the conclusions that have been drawn from this evidence are somewhat controversial. In brief, the evidence for biological theories can be grouped into two main categories: (1) brain morphology/circuitry differences in individuals with and without OCD and, (2) a chemical imbalance in one of the neurotransmitters in the brain of individuals with OCD.

With regard to brain morphology/circuitry differences, some data (e.g., Grados, 2003) suggest that traumatic brain injury (TBI) has a causal role in OCD development. Other data (e.g., Kader, Esmach, Nagy, & Hatata, 2013) suggest a higher frequency of neurological "soft signs" (e.g., abnormal motor or sensory findings and deficits in nonverbal memory and certain executive functions such as set shifting ability, response inhibition, and decision making) in patients diagnosed with OCD. In addition, data suggest structural and functional abnormalities of the brain play a causal role in OCD. For example, the orbitofrontal-subcortical circuits, as seen via positron emission tomography (PET) scans of the orbitofrontal cortex, appear different in patients with and without OCD (Saxena & Rauch, 2000). These circuits are theorized to connect regions of the brain involved in processing of information with regions involved in the initiation of certain behavioral responses, with their hyperactivity hypothesized as leading to the development of OCD symptoms (Breiter et al., 1996; Cottraux et al., 1996). Unfortunately, because these models are only cross-sectional (i.e., occurring at a specific point in time—either before or after the presence of the disorder), it is impossible to determine in a causal manner whether it is the hyperactivity of the circuits that leads to the development of OCD or whether it is the presence of OCD that causes these circuits to become hyperactive.

Researchers (e.g., Barr, Goodman, & Price, 1993) who propose that OCD is caused by a chemical imbalance have traditionally suggested that an inadequate supply of serotonin in turn causes the receptors in the brain that are responsible for metabolizing serotonin to compensate for the low levels by becoming more sensitive, which then somehow plays a causal role in OCD. The serotonin hypothesis was originally generated based on the finding that certain antidepressant medications that block the natural loss of serotonin reduced some of the symptoms in patients diagnosed with OCD. Although this theory has gained some support over the years, it has also been criticized heavily (e.g., Abramowitz & Houts, 2002), on various grounds, including (1) some patients taking drugs impacting serotonin levels do not improve; (2) no data exist to support a relationship between amount of medication taken and degree of symptom relief; (3) older medications that do not increase serotonin levels as well can be as—or more—effective than newer, superior serotonin targeting medications; (4) hypothesizing the cause of a disorder based on the efficacy of a treatment represents an error in logic called the ex post facto fallacy (i.e., that serotonin level enhancers can reduce OCD symptoms does not necessarily mean that the disorder was caused by a shortage of serotonin, in the same way that finding aspirin relieves headaches does not mean headaches are caused by a shortage of aspirin in the brain); (5) treatments not directly targeting serotonin levels (e.g., other classes of medications and nonpharmacological treatments such as

CBT) have been shown to produce equal or superior results; and finally (6) people with OCD have serotonin levels that differ from those of people suffering from other anxiety disorders, or even levels that are different from those of people without any psychological disorder. Therefore, more research is needed to determine the extent to which serotonin functioning mediates OCD symptoms.

Other neurotransmitters that have been hypothesized to play a role in OCD over the years include dopamine (e.g., Kim et al., 2003; Denys, Zohar, & Westenberg, 2004) and glutamate (Pittenger, Bloch, & Williams, 2011). As has been the case with serotonin, however, the precise role of these neurotransmitters in OCD remains unclear, and definitive evidence supporting (or contradicting) them has been slow to emerge (Pittenger et al., 2011). As a result, more, well-controlled studies are needed before the role of neurotransmitters such as these can be understood.

# UNDERSTANDING OCD IN COGNITIVE–BEHAVIORAL TERMS

Starting from the time of Freud, many different psychological theories have been offered in an attempt to explain the etiology and maintenance of OCD. At this time, however, the theories with the most empirical support are behavioral and cognitive theories. Therefore, each of these theories, along with the theories behind two newer approaches that have been gaining empirical support (metacognitive therapy and acceptance and commitment therapy), will be reviewed next.

## Behavioral Theory

The behavioral theory of OCD suggests that people with OCD start to associate certain objects or situations with fear (i.e., classical conditioning) and then learn to either avoid these triggers or perform rituals in order to manage their fears (i.e., operant conditioning). Behavioral theory asserts that the symptoms typically begin during or after stressful life events (Rosso, Asinari, Bogettor, & Maina, 2012), such as moving to a new city, starting a new phase in life (e.g., school, job, relationship), coming to the end of a significant relationship (e.g., the death of a loved one, the break-up of a romantic relationship), or in some cases, after experiencing a severe trauma (de Silva & Marks, 1999).

According to behavioral theory, during these stressful and anxious times, anxiety can generalize to additional, previously neutral stimuli, causing the number of triggers to broaden and thus appear with greater frequency, intensity, and duration over time. Once a connection is established between a trigger and feelings of anxiety, people with OCD either begin to avoid these triggers or learn to engage in both overt and covert rituals in an attempt to neutralize the thoughts, images, and urges and/or decrease the anxiety caused by them. Because these rituals and avoidances work in the short term to reduce anxiety, they become negatively reinforced (i.e., strengthened), which increases the likelihood that they will be utilized in similar situations in the future. In addition, because the rituals are effective in the short term, the individual never feels compelled to learn other, more effective, coping strategies that would actually reduce their anxiety in the long term. However, the price they pay for the short-term relief is that over time, they are forced to engage in more and more rituals in order to reduce their discomfort.

## Cognitive Theory

Whereas the behavioral theory of OCD focuses on how people with OCD make associations between triggers and anxiety, the cognitive theory of OCD focuses on how people with OCD misinterpret their thoughts. The cognitive theory emphasizes the fact that it is common and normal for people to experience the same types of intrusive thoughts as those experienced by people with OCD. What's different, however, is that although most people without OCD may be able to dismiss such thoughts, individuals who are vulnerable to developing OCD misinterpret the intrusive thoughts in certain maladaptive ways. In other words, the cognitive model proposes that it is not the intrusive thoughts per se that generate the strong and unwanted feelings of discomfort or anxiety and urges to ritualize that are the hallmark of OCD, but rather it is what the individual *believes* about the intrusive thoughts that matters.

In 2002, the Obsessive–Compulsive Cognitions Working Group (OCCWG), an international workgroup of researchers interested in the cognitions of patients with OCD, published a book that included several categories of misappraisals (i.e., beliefs) that their research demonstrated as important in the development and maintenance of obsessions. The categories included (1) overestimations of threat; (2) inflated perceptions of personal responsibility; (3) overestimations of the personal significance (i.e., importance) of thoughts, including a concept called thought–action fusion; (4) intolerance of uncertainty; (5) an inflated need for control over thoughts, and (6) an intolerance for the anxiety caused by the thoughts.

According to cognitive theory, these misinterpretations of the thoughts allow the thoughts to gain special importance and in turn, become generators of anxiety and/or other negative emotions, such as shame and guilt. As a result, people with OCD make special efforts to suppress the thoughts, which in turn causes a cascade of insidious effects, including, paradoxically, an increase in thought frequency, a hypervigilance to the thoughts and thought processes, prevention of new learning about the thought's importance, and enhancement of the negative appraisal of the thought's meaning due to inevitable thought recurrences that occur during suppression attempts (Purdon, 2004; Purdon & Clark, 2001). Increased frequency and enhanced negative appraisals induce a more negative mood, which then makes negative thoughts and appraisals more accessible and in turn causes people to try harder to control the thought, neutralize, or cope with the thoughts, ultimately leading to the development of OCD.

## Metacognitive Theory

*Metacognition* is a general term that can be broken down into three main areas (Flavell, 1979; Wells, 2000): metacognitive knowledge, metacognitive experiences, and metacognitive strategies (Rees & Anderson, 2013). Metacognitive knowledge refers to information stored in memory in a declarative form—including false declarative beliefs (i.e., negative metacognitive beliefs). In OCD, an example of a negative metacognitive belief would be that checking rituals protect one's family from harm. Metacognitive experiences refer to the experiences of the OCD patient who might report the feeling of "just knowing," which he or she then uses to guide subsequent actions such as refraining from or completing a ritual (Rees & Anderson, 2013). Metacognitive strategies refer to strategies that people use to regulate and control cognition (e.g., the effort a patient with OCD might make to suppress an unwanted thought).

Wells's (2000) general metacognitive model proposes that a style of thinking called the cognitive attentional syndrome (CAS) is the main causal factor in prolonging all emotional disorders. According to Wells, the CAS consists of three, overlapping components: (1) a perseverative thinking style characterized by worry and rumination; (2) unhelpful hypervigilance for threat; and (3) counterproductive coping which prevents regulation of cognition.

Rees and Anderson (2013) describe nicely how Wells has gone on to specify which aspects of the general metacognitive model are most relevant to understanding OCD:

> Wells (2000) proposes that intrusive thoughts activate negative metacognitive beliefs (metacognitive knowledge) that lead to the CAS. The negative metacognitive beliefs concern the dangerousness and significance of intrusive thoughts (Fisher, 2009). Indeed, Wells argues that three types of metacognitive knowledge are important in the etiology and maintenance of symptoms: thought fusion beliefs, beliefs about the need to perform rituals, and criteria that signal rituals can be stopped. In this model, thought fusion beliefs are extended beyond thought–action fusion (the belief that having a thought increases the chance of acting on it) to also include thought–event fusion (the belief that having a thought can cause an event or means that an event has happened) and thought–object fusion (the belief that thoughts or feelings can be transferred into objects). According to the model, the three overall types of metacognitive knowledge operate in a causal chain to explain obsessive–compulsive symptoms.

Therefore, similar to the cognitive therapy approach for OCD, the main approach in metacognitive therapy of OCD is to help individuals become aware of their metacognitive processing in order to learn to modify their "thoughts about their thoughts" such as beliefs about the dangerousness and significance of thoughts. Where metacognitive therapy differs from cognitive therapy, however, is that the focus is on altering the patient's relationship with their thoughts, as opposed to challenging the "lower-order" appraisals of their thoughts (e.g., "I am responsible to ensure nothing happens to my family"). In other words, metacognitive theory focuses on thinking *processes*. In addition, metacognitive therapy does not emphasize or utilize the habituation strategies found in most behavioral therapies for OCD (e.g., Ex/RP). Instead, individuals typically complete very brief (e.g., 5-minute) "behavioral experiments" designed to assist in the interruption of unhelpful metacognitive processes such as attempts to suppress thoughts (Fisher, 2009).

## Relational Frame Theory

The therapeutic techniques used in acceptance and commitment therapy (ACT; Hayes, Strosahl, & Wilson, 2012) are guided by a philosophy of science called functional contextualism and are informed by behavior analysis and research on language and cognition called relational frame theory (Twohig, 2009). Much like in behavioral theory, relational frame theory views actions as occurring in a three-term contingency consisting of an antecedent (stimulus), a response/behavior, and a consequence. Unlike behavioral theory, however, relational frame theory does not assert that experience with the antecedents or consequences are required for them to acquire functions. Instead, relational frame theory posits that our ability to respond relationally allows stimuli to acquire functions without experience.

According to relational frame theory, people learn how to transfer the functions of stimuli to other stimuli using a variety of frames, including similarity, opposition, distinction, comparison, hierarchy, time, space, causality, and relationship and perspective (Twohig, 2009). For example, if a person with contamination-type OCD experiences "dirty" things as dangerous, anything similar to "dirty" will acquire the functions of "dangerous." As a result, many arbitrary stimuli can acquire fearful and anxiety-provoking functions even though a person has no experience with them. This is particularly important because it shows that processes other than our interaction with our environment influence our behavior and lead to behaviors that are inconsistent with environmental contingencies and are instead guided by cognitive contingencies (Twohig, 2009).

Behavior guided by cognitive contingencies (i.e., not learned through interaction with the environment) can be problematic, however, because (1) the behavior may not change when the actual or real-world contingencies change; and (2) the contingency specified may be incorrect (i.e., because of our cognitive abilities, we can respond to contingencies that are only in our heads and not necessarily related to the way the world really works). Thus, although cognitive abilities are useful in most situations, they can become too dominant.

Twohig (2009) describes how cognitive contingencies can be problematic in OCD:

> Cognitive abilities provide two beliefs that support pathology: (a) negatively evaluated inner experiences are dangerous; (b) negatively evaluated inner experiences need to be diminished or controlled. It is sometimes useful to regulate emotions, but this is not a rule to be applied in all situations. In fact, attempting to control or regulate obsessions (and associated anxiety or fear) is largely what makes OCD a disorder. Support for conceptualizing OCD as a disorder of misplaced rules regarding danger-ous inner experiences that should be controlled comes from the diagnostic criteria for OCD (Ameri-can Psychiatric Association, 2013), and from self-reports of people diagnosed with OCD in which 90% admit that compulsions are performed to reduce distress from obsessions (Foa & Kozak, 1995). Attempts to suppress obsessions are generally not effective (Purdon, 2004; Purdon & Clark, 2001), and a key component of effective treatments for OCD involve[s] exposure and reduction of neutralizing responses (Abramowitz, 1996). Finally, attempts at regulating these inner experiences (e.g., compul-sions) backfire and result in reduced rather than increased quality of life (e.g., Koran, Theinemann, & Davenport, 1996). OCD is pretty clearly a case where the cognitive contingency is very different than the real-world one. (p. 19)

ACT, like CBT, targets avoidance—only in this case its target is "experiential" avoidance, which is defined as when "a person is unwilling to remain in contact with particular private experiences and takes steps to alter the form or frequency of these events and the contexts that occasion them—even when attempts to do so negatively affect quality of life" (Hayes, Wilson, Gif-ford, Follette, & Strosahl, 1996, p. 1154). However, ACT does not address any specific cognitions, emotions, or physiological sensations. Instead, the treatment targets both the *cognitive contingency* in which they occur and the patient's *responses* to these cognitive experiences. This approach is based on the notion that once the dominance of the cognitive contingency is reduced, the patient can be in greater contact with the real-world contingencies that shape more functional behavior.

In addition to reducing the dominance of the cognitive contingency, ACT also focuses on helping individuals to commit to move in a direction in life that is meaningful to them. As such, ACT also differs from cognitive and behavioral models of OCD in that it emphasizes that it is not necessary to wait for a decrease in obsessive thoughts and/or anxiety in order to begin changing one's actions and move forward in directions that are meaningful. In other words, from an ACT point of view, OCD's negative impact is not necessarily caused by the presence of obsessions and compulsions; rather, it is due to the fact that every time an obsessive thought is experienced, the person chooses to respond by engaging in a compulsion. Therefore, ACT aims to teach the individual how to be flexible in his responses, so that the person learns to see that he has a number of alternative responses to choose from when he experiences an obsession. ACT proposes that regular practice of this method will make it easier to tolerate obsessions and/or feelings of anxiety, and thereby prevent them from interfering with one's life.

---

## TAKE-HOME MESSAGE

OCD is a prevalent and debilitating psychological disorder with a chronic course if left untreated. The disorder can take on many forms, so it is important to understand the various subtypes and be able to differentiate OCD from other disorders. At this time, the exact cause of OCD is unknown, and it is unlikely that a single cause will be identified in the near future. It is safe to say, however, that genetics and biological circuitry, along with the environment (early learning and life stressors), all play a role in the etiology of OCD. As a result, most experts will likely continue to view OCD as a multidetermined disorder, with both biological and psychological factors playing key roles in its etiology and maintenance. In terms of psychological theories, behavioral and cognitive theories, along with metacognitive and relational frame theories, all offer interesting explanations. Fortunately, regardless of the cause, a number of established and promising pharmacological and psychological treatments are available for OCD, which will be covered in the next chapter.

# CHAPTER 3

# Evidence-Based Treatments for Obsessive–Compulsive Disorder

As mentioned in Chapter 2, the exact cause of OCD is unknown, and it is unlikely that a single cause will be identified in the near future. Despite—or perhaps because of—that knowledge gap, a number of promising treatments for OCD have been created and studied, leading to many advances in the treatment of OCD. In fact, as a result of these advances, our entire notion of what it means to have OCD has changed over the past 30–40 years, from that of a diagnosis with a poor prognosis to one in which many individuals can expect to see a significant response to treatment and, occasionally, a full remission of the disorder. Of the many treatments offered for OCD, the ones with the strongest evidence base at this time are cognitive-behavioral therapy and a class of medications called the selective serotonin reuptake inhibitors (SSRIs; e.g., fluoxetine [Prozac], fluvoxamine [Luvox], sertraline [Zoloft], paroxetine [Paxil] and citalopram [Celexa]). I will review these treatments in detail below, followed by a discussion of several additional treatments that have a growing evidence base but are not quite as well established in the treatment outcome literature at this time.

## COGNITIVE-BEHAVIORAL THERAPY

Within the field of CBT, two distinct treatments have each received strong empirical support for reducing the obsessions and compulsions found in OCD: (1) Ex/RP, a specific type of behavioral therapy and (2) cognitive therapy. Although most clinicians offer these treatments in combination, I will discuss them separately, as they stem from different theoretical models (see Chapter 2).

## EXPOSURE AND RITUAL PREVENTION

Ex/RP has the strongest evidence base and is the mostly widely utilized psychosocial treatment for OCD. Ex/RP involves two main components: (1) direct or imagined, controlled exposure to situations, objects, or other triggers of the patient's obsessive thoughts that create anxiety and; (2) prevention of the patient from engaging in any rituals aimed at reducing the anxiety caused by the exposure. These components allow the patient to "habituate" (i.e., "get used to") to the anxiety caused by their obsessions and, through repetition, weaken the connection between experiencing an obsession and needing to engage in a compulsion to neutralize either the thought or the anxiety, or both, that the obsession generated. As a result, over time the patient learns that the anxiety caused by the obsession will diminish on its own and that the feared consequences do not come true. Thus, further exposures to the situations, objects, or other triggers will generate less and less anxiety over time.

Ex/RP is conducted in a structured, hierarchical manner, with items in the hierarchy being arranged according to the level of distress/anxiety the patient anticipates they will cause when faced (patients are typically trained to rate their anxiety levels using a 0–10 or 0–100 scale).[1] Traditionally, the treatment started with the patient confronting an item he anticipated would cause a mild/moderate (e.g., 4/10) level of anxiety. It was argued that starting exposure using an item that generated too little distress/anxiety would prevent the patient's "fear structure" from being activated (i.e., not anxiety-provoking enough, so no new learning about the trigger would occur) while starting with an item that generated too much distress may overwhelm the patient and prevent habituation from occurring (i.e., the patient would be too emotionally flooded to learn anything new about the trigger). Therefore, starting with an item in the mild/moderate range is thought to create the ideal opportunity for new learning and habituation to occur. Then, as the patient habituates to each item, he gradually works up the hierarchy to situations that cause greater and greater levels of anxiety and eventually, to new situations that occur "naturalistically" in his daily life.

Typically, each exposure item is first faced in session, often with the therapist role-modeling and/or assisting in some way. Exposure sessions typically range between 45 and 90 minutes but can last as long as several hours, as traditionally, experts believed that there needed to be enough time for habituation to occur, in order for exposure therapy to be successful. In addition, patients are required to practice Ex/RP between sessions, for at least one or two hours per day, for the item on the hierarchy that was addressed that week (as well as any similarly rated or lower-rated items from previous weeks). The time it takes to move from one item to the next typically depends on a combination of the patient's ability to tolerate anxiety, resist engaging in compulsions, and practice between sessions.

Ideally, Ex/RP is conducted *in vivo* (in "real-life" situations), depending on the particulars of the obsessive thoughts. For example, an *in vivo* exposure exercise might involve leaving the therapist's office, with the patient walking out last and without checking to make sure the door is locked, or walking around the therapist's building and touching various "contaminated" areas and/or objects without engaging in any hand washing during or afterward, and then "spreading" the contamination by having the patient "wipe" his hands over his clothes, hair, and face.

In some cases, however, *in vivo* exposure to the obsessional fears may either be realistically harmful or impossible to create in a session (e.g., fear of murdering a loved one, sexually molesting an innocent victim, contracting AIDS, going to hell). In these cases, Ex/RP is conducted using *imaginal exposure* (i.e., vividly imagining the obsessive thought/scenario in detail, including aversive consequences, in the here-and-now and without neutralizing it in any way). For example, a patient with an obsession about murdering a loved one would be asked to create a scenario in which the worst case (i.e., murder of the loved one) occurs, along with the consequences (e.g., going to jail,

---

[1]Recently, some researchers (e.g., Craske et al., 2012) have called this notion into question.

being disowned by family, being shunned by society), and then rehearse it repeatedly—either by writing it out over and over again or by recording it and then listening to it each day.

In some cases, the fear may be activated by a single sentence ("I'm going to murder my wife" or "I've hit and killed a pedestrian"). In these cases, the patient may write the sentence out over and over again while picturing the scene. Or the patient may record the sentence and play it back, over and over (modern digital recorders and smart phones with voice memos are great for this). In some cases, the most anxiety-provoking situation may be one in which the patient is uncertain of the outcome, as opposed to the worst-case outcome (e.g., "I *may* have contracted AIDS" vs. "I *have* contracted AIDS"). For some patients, not knowing (i.e., having to tolerate uncertainty) feels worse than knowing, even if the outcome is negative. In these cases, the imaginal exposure exercises would have to be adjusted accordingly.

Regardless of whether you use *in vivo* or imaginal exposure, the main goal is for the patient to remain in contact with the situation, object, or trigger of the obsessions, without engaging in any rituals to "neutralize" the anxiety or thoughts in any way. Understandably, undergoing exposure without being allowed to perform rituals is a challenging task for nearly all patients—especially at the beginning of treatment. As a result, in order to maintain patient rapport and motivation, when starting Ex/RP many therapists collaborate with the patient to set up a minimum period of time for ritual prevention and then gradually increase period of time as treatment progresses. For example, the patient with contamination fears whose first task is to walk around the therapist's building and touch various "contaminated" objects may initially be asked just to engage in ritual prevention (e.g., resist hand washing) immediately after the session and, if he needs to wash, to use a quick, cold-water rinse instead of hot water and soap. In subsequent exposures, however, the patient may be asked to resist washing for several hours and eventually for days after an exposure task—all while still engaging in otherwise "normal" daily activities. The therapy continues in this way until the patient is able to resist engaging in rituals altogether while living the life she wants to live (i.e., she returns to "normal" functioning).

## COGNITIVE THERAPY

Cognitive therapy for OCD, which stems from the cognitive theory of OCD (see Chapter 2), targets the maladaptive *appraisals* of intrusive thoughts that are believed to lead to the development and maintenance of OCD. Recall that it is normal for people *without* a diagnosis of OCD to experience the *exact same intrusive thought*s as those experienced by patients diagnosed with OCD. As a result, the cognitive model suggests that rather than the content of the thoughts, what's different is that patients diagnosed with OCD *misinterpret their thoughts* in certain problematic ways (i.e., make *maladaptive appraisals*), which leads them to become anxious and perform rituals and ultimately turn what are commonly experienced intrusive thoughts into actual obsessions.

For example, an atheist and a devoutly religious person may both experience the same intrusive thought about committing a sacrilegious or blasphemous act. Theoretically, however, the atheist would be less likely to react to the intrusive thought with a significant increase in anxiety because she would be less likely than a devoutly religious person to appraise it as negatively. As a result, the devoutly religious person will become very anxious and will be more likely to ritualize in some way to relieve the distress caused by the intrusive thought.

Thus, cognitive theory asserts that it is not intrusive thoughts that generate the strong and unwanted feelings of discomfort or anxiety and urges to ritualize that are the hallmark of OCD, but rather the patient's *maladaptive appraisals* of the intrusive thoughts. As a result, cognitive therapy aims to help patients identify, challenge, and modify the maladaptive beliefs (i.e., appraisals) they hold about their obsessive thoughts. In other words, cognitive therapy focuses on correcting how patients *interpret* (i.e., react to) their obsessions, including why they think they have the obsessions, what they believe having the obsessions says about them, and what their attitude is toward them (in terms of importance, control, etc.).

This change is achieved through various common cognitive techniques. These include psychoeducation, in which a therapist (1) describes obsessions as ordinary intrusions experienced by everyone; (2) teaches patients about the cognitive model of OCD; (3) engages the patient in Socratic dialogues about the contributions of early experience, mood, and core beliefs to the interpretation of intrusive thoughts; and (4) assigns homework in which the patient monitors and records her triggers, obsessive thoughts, maladaptive appraisals, and rituals.

Cognitive techniques can also be used to target specific OCD-related appraisals (e.g., inflated responsibility, intolerance of uncertainty, perfectionism, importance of thoughts) that correspond with the patient's obsessive thoughts. Note once again that the treatment does not attempt to address the obsessions (e.g., fear of committing a violent act directly) but rather targets the maladaptive appraisals (e.g., "Having this thought is important" or "I should be in control of my thoughts at all times") that are associated with the obsessions. This difference is critically important, for attempting to target the obsessions directly may increase their importance, which may then lead patients to pay more attention to them and notice them more frequently (i.e., increase their obsessing).

The specific cognitive techniques and strategies used to challenge and correct the maladaptive appraisals may include cognitive restructuring exercises, such as (1) calculating the probability of harm when patients overestimate the likelihood of danger; (2) using the "pie" technique to address inflated responsibility; and (3) employing Socratic dialogue to examine the evidence for appraisals that appear flawed. In addition, cognitive therapy may include using the "downward-arrow" technique to identify and modify core beliefs, and even employ mindfulness training to teach patients how to observe and then distance themselves from their intrusive thoughts and thus tolerate them better. These techniques are described in greater detail in Chapter 14.

Cognitive therapy also utilizes behavioral experiments, both during and between sessions, to encourage a shift in attitude by helping patients learn to test out their hypotheses. Although on the surface these experiments may appear similar to the exposure techniques of Ex/RP, in cognitive therapy typically they are fairly brief and do not focus on habituation to discomfort/distress. Although some researchers (e.g., Sookman & Steketee, 2007) have suggested that the use of behavioral experiments to test hypotheses may render cognitive therapy less threatening and more acceptable to some patients than Ex/RP, in clinical practice, cognitive therapy techniques are often used in conjunction with Ex/RP.

## A SCHEMA-BASED MODEL

Sookman and colleagues (Sookman, Pinard, & Beauchemin, 1994; Sookman & Pinaud, 1999, 2007) have also developed and elaborated a schema-based conceptual and treatment approach for OCD of different subtypes. Sookman and Steketee (2007) note that the rationale for using this approach comes from Rosen (1989), who states that dysfunctional schemas may interfere with learning during basic cognitive therapy because they do not accommodate disconfirmatory experiences. For example, the core belief "I am a vulnerable or dangerous person" could influence the appraisal of thoughts and other strategic processing of inner and external events.

Sookman and Steketee (2007) assert that dysfunctional schemas may underlie intransigent emotional beliefs about threat (Sookman & Pinard, 2002) and risk aversion (Steketee & Frost, 1994) in patients who are unable to engage fully in Ex/RP (Sookman & Pinard, 2007). According to contemporary CBT models, (1) dysfunctional responses to internal and external events are manifestations of dysfunction at the core schema level, and (2) modification of the structure and content of dysfunctional schemas is necessary to forestall recurrence of symptoms (Beck, 1996). Thus, they conclude that treatment with CBT to modify these symptoms requires an integrative, schema-based approach.

In the schema-based approach of Sookman and colleagues, schema-based interventions are used to broaden the scope of cognitive therapy in order to increase participation in Ex/RP, improve maintenance and generalization of change, and reduce susceptibility to relapse (Sookman & Steketee, 2007). These interventions are typically combined with (1) traditional cognitive therapy techniques (to modify appraisals and beliefs and reduce anxiety), (2) intensive Ex/RP (to reduce rituals), (3) behavioral experiments (to foster disconfirmatory learning), and (4) techniques for developing new skills.

## COGNITIVE THERAPY VERSUS BEHAVIORAL THERAPY

To date, there have only been a handful of controlled studies comparing cognitive therapy with Ex/RP for patients with OCD (e.g., van Oppen et al., 1995; Cottraux et al., 2001; McLean et al., 2001; Whittal, Thordarson & McLean, 2005). As a result of this paucity of available data, it is difficult to draw any firm conclusions about the comparative efficacy of these two treatments. Nevertheless, it does appear safe to say that both treatments lead to similar and significant pre–post improvements, which are generally maintained through follow-up periods. In addition, two interesting trends have emerged. First, although both treatments appear to be effective for OCD when delivered individually, it appears that cognitive therapy may be a more effective choice in individual cases where Ex/RP is difficult to apply (e.g., with "pure obsessionals" who deny engaging in any form of compulsion). Second, Ex/RP appears to do equally well in both individual and group modalities and to outperform cognitive therapy in a group therapy modality.

## GROUP CBT FOR OCD

By offering CBT in a group modality, therapists trained in CBT can reach more individuals with OCD at once, which could help dissemination efforts by reducing wait lists. In addition, group treatments tend to be relatively less expensive than individual treatments, as most group therapists reduce the per patient fee, in part as an incentive for patients to join and in part because of the less concentrated attention each member receives. As mentioned above, there is growing support in the literature for the efficacy and effectiveness of group CBT that employs Ex/RP for OCD. Most studies show that group treatment for OCD generally demonstrates results that are equivalent to individual treatment in terms of reduction of obsessions and compulsions; some data even suggest that the group approach may enhance compliance with treatment. At present, however, group CBT remains a second-line treatment, according to various expert consensus guidelines (e.g., March, Frances, Carpenter, & Kahn, 1997; National Institute for Health and Clinical Excellence, 2005; Nathan & Gorman, 2015; *www.psychologicaltreatments.org*).

## MEDICATIONS FOR OCD

Experts have recognized a number of medications as effective in reducing the obsessions and compulsions found in OCD. In addition, these medications can be particularly useful for patients diagnosed with OCD and comorbid depression. At this time, expert consensus guidelines (e.g., March et al., 1997; National Institute for Health and Clinical Excellence, 2005; Nathan and Gorman, 2007; *www.psychologicaltreatments.org*) recommend six medications as first-line treatments for OCD: fluvoxamine (Luvox), fluoxetine (Prozac), sertraline (Zoloft), paroxetine (Paxil), citalopram (Celexa), and clomipramine (Anafranil). Of these, the first five medications are hypothesized to selectively target the reuptake of the neurotransmitter serotonin. They are considered to be safer and have fewer side effects than the older antidepressant medications (such as clomipramine, which is in the class of medications called the tricyclic antidepressants).

## CBT VERSUS MEDICATIONS FOR OCD

Given that strong evidence supports both CBT and medications in the treatment of OCD, a question that often arises is how well they fare when compared head-to-head. Studies directly comparing their relative efficacy have generally been methodologically complex but appear to yield equivocal results: at posttreatment, both treatments appear to be superior to placebo, with Ex/RP showing results superior to medications and the combination of the two treatments not being superior to Ex/RP alone (e.g., Foa et al., 2005). In addition, relapse appears to be more evident following the discontinuation of medications than in Ex/RP and the combination of the two treatments (e.g., Simpson et al., 2004).

Perhaps as a result of these findings, the OCD Expert Consensus Guidelines strongly recommend starting with CBT, either alone or combined with pharmacotherapy, as the first-line treatment. Either way, however, it is important to be familiar with—and to share as part of informed consent procedures—the following pros and cons of each treatment.

For medications, the pros include the fact that they (1) require less effort than engaging in CBT (no daily homework, etc.); (2) are more widely available/easier to access than CBT (it remains difficult to find a therapist properly trained to do Ex/RP); (3) appear to be more helpful in addressing symptoms such as pathological doubt and aggressive obsessions, as well as mental rituals for slowness, hoarding, and tic-like symptoms; and (4) are relatively safe.

Some of the cons of medications include the fact that they (1) will only produce a positive response ("much" or "very much" improved on clinical global impression ratings) in approximately 40–60% of patients, with many patients continuing to experience residual symptoms; (2) often produce unpleasant side effects (e.g., gastrointestinal distress, restlessness, insomnia, and sexual dysfunction), especially given the fact that the treatment guidelines suggest that dosing trials for

OCD with the SSRIs should typically be at higher doses and for a longer duration than doses for the other anxiety disorders and depression; (3) must be continually taken in order to maintain treatment gains; leading them to (4) be more costly than CBT in the long term and/or (5) show a higher relapse rate than CBT once discontinued.

Unlike medications, CBT using Ex/RP produces (1) an equal or greater decrease in OCD symptoms in a treatment package that is (2) relatively brief in duration, and (3) has a greater durability (i.e., much lower relapse rate than medications), and (4) without any side effects (unless one counts the short-term increase in anxiety as patients engage in the Ex/RP portion of the treatment). The cons of CBT, however, include the fact that it (1) remains difficult to find and access therapists who have been trained to deliver the treatment, (2) requires the patient to work hard— within and between the sessions—to be effective, and (3) has a high rejection rate from patients.

## WHICH TO START WITH: CBT OR MEDICATIONS?

Given the above data, expert consensus guidelines (e.g., March et al., 1997; National Institute for Health and Clinical Excellence, 2005; Nathan & Gorman, 2015; *www.psychologicaltreatments.org*) usually suggest beginning the treatment of OCD patients with either CBT alone or a combination of CBT and a medication. According to expert consensus guidelines, the likelihood that medication will be included in the recommendation varies with the severity of the OCD and the age of the patient. For example, in milder OCD, CBT alone is the expert consensus initial choice. As severity increases, however, the experts are more likely to suggest adding medication to CBT as the initial treatment or to use medication alone. Finally, in younger patients, the experts are more likely to suggest using CBT alone.

## COMBINING CBT AND MEDICATIONS

Although both CBT and pharmacotherapy have strong empirical support for their clinical efficacy and effectiveness, both also frequently leave symptoms remaining at posttreatment. In other words, often no true "cure" is possible, and, under the best of circumstances, patients receiving either one of the two, expert consensus treatments of choice for OCD will still be symptomatic at posttreatment (i.e., show a "response" to treatment but not achieve full remission of symptoms). Perhaps as a result of this finding, many mental health professionals advocate for *combining* CBT with pharmacotherapy to "maximize" treatment outcome.

Unfortunately and interestingly, very few studies have tested this idea. The limited number of studies examining combination therapy for OCD have generally found that at posttreatment and follow-up there was no demonstrable advantage or disadvantage of combined treatment over *intensive* CBT delivered alone (e.g., Otto, Smits, & Reese, 2006). In contrast to this finding, however, the data suggest that combined treatment may have some advantage over *medications* alone. This finding has led some researchers (e.g., Foa, Franklin, & Moser, 2002) to suggest adding CBT to the treatment of patients who initially received medications alone. In addition, as mentioned above, the combination has also been suggested as being useful to manage any comorbid syndromes that are known to negatively impact Ex/RP outcome, such as major depressive disorder, as well as when the OCD is more severe. What remains to be established, however, is the optimal sequencing of these treatments (Franklin & Foa, 2011).

## OTHER OPTIONS FOR TREATMENT–REFRACTORY PATIENTS (PARTIAL RESPONDERS AND NONRESPONDERS)

Although the expert consensus is quite clear that CBT, the SSRIs or both should be the first-line interventions for OCD, there is somewhat less expert consensus about what to do next when managing patients who remain symptomatic after receiving well-delivered CBT and/or a trial on an SSRI (i.e., treatment-refractory patients). With regard to CBT, researchers have been exploring variations in the level of care. For example, although the expert consensus guidelines recommend beginning CBT with 13–20 weekly, individual CBT sessions and note that standard treatment should also employ between-session homework assignments and therapist-assisted out-of-office (i.e., *in vivo*) Ex/RP, they also assert that when the OCD is particularly severe, more intensive CBT may be preferable.

For example, some treatment protocols have studied the efficacy of CBT for OCD when administered in either twice-weekly or daily sessions of up to 90–120 minutes. Interestingly, the data suggest that five Ex/RP sessions delivered per week may be more effective than once-weekly sessions, but are not necessarily any more effective than sessions delivered twice per week. So far, though, the optimal number of treatment sessions, as well as their length, and the duration of an adequate trial have not yet been definitively established in the literature.

Expert consensus guidelines suggest that although outpatient treatment is usually sufficient for OCD (and is consistent with the notion that treatment should generally be provided in the least restrictive setting that is both safe and effective), there are times when a more intensive treatment setting may be indicated.[2] The following factors should be considered when determining the appropriate setting for treatment: in the presence of risk to life, severe self-neglect, and extreme distress or functional impairment. For each of these factors, the expert consensus guidelines provide indications for a more intense setting, including the initiation of home-based treatment, partial hospitalization, residential treatment, and inpatient treatment. Thus, when you assess a patient and find that he presents with one or more of these factors, a referral is appropriate—either to a clinic that is set up to provide more frequent or longer sessions, or to an appropriate inpatient facility with expertise in treating OCD, as once-weekly "dosing" may not be sufficient to make an impact on the disorder.

For example, inpatient services may be necessary for patients who cannot provide adequate self-care, are not able to engage in consistent ritual prevention, or are restricting their eating due to their obsessions, as well as for patients who have a significant comorbid condition (e.g., major depression, schizophrenia, or mania) that is negatively impacting the treatment. Residential treat-

---

[2]In keeping with this "stepped-care" model, conversely, some patients (e.g., those assessed to have a mild form of OCD) may benefit from simply a good self-help book suggestion (e.g., *Stop Obsessing!: How to Overcome Your Obsessions and Compulsions* [Foa & Wilson, 2001] or *Overcoming Obsessive Thoughts: How to Gain Control of Your OCD* [Purdon & Clark, 2005]; see Appendix A) without needing to see a therapist and others may need only a slightly more intense treatment, such as a guided self-help model (e.g., having the patient work through a self-help book with occasional visits to the therapist for assistance).

ment may be indicated in individuals with severe treatment-resistant OCD, who require multidisciplinary treatment in a highly structured setting that permits intensive individual and group CBT as well as psychopharmacologic management. Partial hospitalization may be indicated by a need for daily CBT and monitoring of behavior or medications or a supportive milieu with other adjunctive psychosocial interventions, or to stabilize and increase the gains made during a period of full hospitalization. Home-based treatment may be necessary initially for those with contamination fears or other symptoms so impairing that they cannot come to the office or clinic. Finally, home-based treatment may also be indicated for individuals who experience symptoms primarily or exclusively at home.

With regard to medication options, as a first step, the expert consensus guidelines recommend that psychiatrists gradually increase the dose of the SSRI to its maximum within 4–8 weeks from the start of treatment for individuals showing an initial nonresponse to the average dose, and to gradually increase the dose to its maximum within 5–9 weeks from the start of treatment for individuals showing only a partial response to the average dose. The guidelines also state that a few patients who show only a partial response to medication but few side effects may benefit from doses substantially higher than those listed as the conventional maximum. They caution, however, that the dose of medication for such patients should not be increased to high levels until at least 12 weeks of treatment have elapsed.

Expert consensus guidelines also suggest that after a patient has had an adequate medication trial for 8–13 weeks, either changing medications or augmenting the initial medication with another medication should be considered. The experts suggest a variety of augmentation strategies that can be tried in patients with OCD, including switching to the tricyclic antidepressant clomipramine. This medication arguably has an efficacy rate that is near equivalent to the SSRIs but was bumped to the last of the six "first-line" recommendations because it produces a broader range of side effects and is less safe in the event of an overdose. In addition, medications from other classes of drugs have been suggested, such as using a benzodiazepine, conventional neuroleptics, buspirone, risperidone, and even a second SSRI to augment the first one.

Expert consensus guidelines suggest tailoring the choice of augmentation medications to the individual clinical presentation. For example, they suggest that clomipramine may be useful in boosting the response of a patient treated with an SSRI who is not having an adequate response; that a neuroleptic may be helpful for patients who are not having an adequate response to an SRI and who have a comorbid tic disorder, OCD symptoms that resemble tics, or comorbid schizotypy; and that a benzodiazepine may be helpful for patients with a comorbid anxiety disorder. Other treatments, including venlafaxine and the monoamine oxidase inhibitors (MAOIs), are seen as third-line treatments and are only to be considered in patients in whom SSRIs and clomipramine have not proven helpful. Finally, the expert consensus guidelines also note that though little empirical documentation exists, case studies and open trials support the same augmentation strategies for pediatric as for adult patients.

## D-CYCLOSERINE

A relatively recent development in the treatment of anxiety disorders has been to augment CBT with D-cycloserine (DCS), an old antibiotic medication originally designed for the treatment of tuberculosis. Rather than being hypothesized to work based on the notion that some underlying neurochemical or neurophysiological abnormalities exist that need to be corrected, DCS is thought to work by indirectly increasing glutamatergic transmission in the N-methyl-D-aspartate (NMDA) receptors in the amygdala. DCS, a partial NMDA receptor agonist, is hypothesized to enhance the learning process underlying extinction of fear either by enhancing NMDA receptor function during extinction or by reducing NMDA receptor function during fear memory consolidation. In other words, researchers propose that DCS will work by enhancing the "emotional learning" (or unlearning, as the case may be in exposure) that occurs with CBT, rather than correct a chemical (e.g., serotonin) imbalance in the brain.

Strong evidence exists to support DCS as an enhancer of fear extinction in animals. Preliminary evidence is mounting to suggest that it can do the same (when used with exposure therapy) in people with anxiety disorders—including acrophobia, social phobia, panic disorder, and OCD. Currently, DCS appears to be more effective when administered (1) a limited number of times and (2) immediately before or after a session focusing on exposure. In general, thus far the major contribution of DCS to exposure-based therapy is thought to be that it can increase the speed or efficiency of CBT, as the effects of DCS seem to decrease over repeated sessions. In addition, the gains made in treatment are generally maintained at follow-up, although some deterioration of gains has been reported.

Specifically with regard to OCD, a study by Kushner et al. (2007) examined DCS as an augmentation strategy for Ex/RP in 32 patients diagnosed with OCD. The study found that, in comparison to a placebo control, participants who received twice-weekly exposure and response prevention plus 10 doses of 125 milligrams of DCS were less likely to discontinue the therapy and required fewer exposure sessions to achieve a 50% reduction in distress from baseline. In addition, after four exposure sessions, patients in the DCS group reported significantly greater decreases in obsession-related distress as compared with the placebo group. These results were in accordance with a study by Wilhelm et al. (2008), which together suggest that acute administration of DCS can facilitate the effects of Ex/RP for OCD. Obviously, more research is needed on this exciting and promising development in the treatment of OCD.

## OTHER PSYCHOLOGICAL TREATMENTS

### Metacognitive Therapy

As mentioned in Chapter 2, metacognitive therapy for OCD aims to help patients become aware of their metacognitive processing so that they can learn to modify their metacognitions (i.e., thoughts about their thoughts), such as beliefs that certain thoughts are more important than others and/or dangerous to think. As such, the focus in metacognitive therapy is on helping the patient alter his relationship with his thoughts, instead of attempting to challenge the thoughts or appraisals he may have of them. In addition, metacognitive therapy does not employ Ex/RP, but rather has patients conduct brief behavioral experiments that are typically created to assist in the interruption of unhelpful metacognitive processes. Although studies evaluating the efficacy of metacognitive therapy for OCD are in their infancy (e.g., only three small-scale studies), the results are promising and warrant further large-scale investigations (Fisher, 2009).

### Acceptance and Commitment Therapy

ACT, like metacognitive therapy, does not directly address specific cognitions. Instead, the treatment aims to teach patients how to be flexible in the way they respond to their thoughts and emotions. In so doing, patients learn that they can choose from a number of alternative responses—other than engaging in a compulsion—when they experience an obsessive thought or feel anxious. ACT also aims to help patients identify the aspects of their lives that are meaningful to them and then teaches them how to commit to pursuing them, despite whatever is going on inside of them (e.g., obsessions, anxiety). Also like metacognitive therapy, the current state of evidence for ACT for OCD is limited (one single case study, one case series, and one controlled study on ACT for OCD) but promising.

## OTHER BIOLOGICAL TREATMENTS

In patients with extremely severe and treatment-refractory OCD who do not respond to any of the interventions suggested above, the expert consensus guidelines suggest that some consideration be given to an IV form of clomipramine. In addition, stereotactic neurological procedures that involve brain surgeries such as cingulotomies and orbitofrontal leukotomies are still being used (often as a last resort, owing to their irreversibility) and have produced improvements in some intransigent cases, but they lack controlled trial data, including long-term follow-up on adverse effects. Finally, although convulsive stimulation (e.g., ECT) is not considered to be effective for OCD (though it may help relieve severe comorbid depression), subconvulsive stimulation treatments (e.g., transcranial magnetic stimulation, vagus nerve stimulation, and deep brain stimulation), which involve less intracerebral neuronal damage, are showing early signs of promise but need more rigorous investigation (Husted & Shapira, 2004).

## A NOTE ON THE INCREASING INTEREST IN THE USE OF VARIOUS TECHNOLOGIES TO DISSEMINATE CBT FOR OCD

As mentioned above, one of the cons of CBT is the fact that the majority of professionals who are trained in it are clustered around major urban areas, while sufferers are dispersed throughout the country—and the world. This dilemma of providing evidence-based mental health services to patients in remote locations has spurred an interest in the study of emerging health information technologies for use in the treatment of OCD using CBT.

These various technologies (e.g., e-mail encryption, real-time chats, webcams, videoconferencing, secure web-based text-messaging services, smart phone applications) are advancing at an increasing pace and have led to the creation of various forms of e-therapy (i.e., Internet-based therapy). The types of e-therapy range from peer-to-peer online support groups to organized services that provide mental health advice online, to fee-based, pay-per-question mental health services that providers answer, to true e-therapy which, using video teleconferencing services (e.g., Skype, FaceTime), aims to establish longer-term, ongoing helping relationships communicating via the Internet.

Although teletherapy clearly poses many potential benefits (e.g., reduce wait lists, cut travel time, improve access), critics have pointed out that it is also not without significant potential risks (e.g., confidentiality, crisis management, legal, ethical, and jurisdictional issues). In addition, research on the efficacy and effectiveness of e-therapy is still in its infancy. As the ethics and legalities of these treatments are clarified, we should expect to see an increase in the study and use of this modality of treatment—as a stand-alone therapy, some form of hybrid treatment (e.g., with patients splitting time between office visits and Internet-based sessions), or even computer-delivered therapy.

---

## TAKE-HOME MESSAGE

Whereas OCD was once considered to be an untreatable disorder, incredible progress has been made over the past few decades on the development and empirical evaluation of treatments for OCD. Presently, the two treatments of choice for OCD are CBT and the SSRIs, with expert consensus guidelines suggesting that the treatment begin with either CBT alone or a combination of CBT and an SSRI. Standard CBT treatment should begin with 13–20 weekly, individual sessions and include between-session assignments and therapist-assisted out-of-office (i.e., *in vivo*) Ex/RP. Variations on this standard starting point for treatment should take into account the severity of the OCD, the age of the patient, if there is risk to life, severe self-neglect, extreme distress or functional impairment, comorbidity, the acceptability of the treatment to the patient, and the like. Several promising new psychological, pharmacological, and biological treatments have also been developed but need more rigorous evaluation at this time. These include metacognitive therapy, ACT, augmentation of CBT with DCS, use of various new technologies, and several stereotactic neurological procedures that involve brain surgeries as well as subconvulsive stimulation treatments.

# CHAPTER 4

# Assessment and Diagnosis

This chapter, along with Chapter 5, will describe everything a clinician will need to do to assess and differentially diagnose OCD, as well as formulate the case for the patient in order to prepare him for treatment. These steps are typically conducted over one or two sessions and include (1) conducting a brief phone screen; (2) completing an intake evaluation (a structured diagnostic interview and a general clinical evaluation); (3) augmenting the evaluation with evidence-based, clinician-administered, OCD-specific assessment measures; (4) assigning a comprehensive, empirically based self-report measures packet for the patient to complete; and (5) giving feedback and presenting a case formulation to the patient.

A careful and detailed assessment and proper case formulation are *both* necessary to increase the likelihood of providing a successful treatment, regardless of whether the treatment is manualized. All too often, novice therapists make the mistake of doing a cursory evaluation to generate a preliminary diagnosis and then believe they can simply fit the patient into a protocol created for that particular diagnosis. Reinforcing this notion is the fact that many protocols, which have been built on a solid, empirically derived conceptual foundation, are robust enough to be effective with less complicated patients. As patients become more diagnostically complex, however, ignoring individual factors such as symptom history and course, motivation, and insight can lead to poor treatment outcome, even with evidence-based treatment protocols. As such, it is wise to gather enough information at the outset of treatment not only to make a diagnosis, but also to aid in making treatment planning decisions (e.g., the most appropriate level of care, whether medications are indicated), as well as facilitate in building rapport and alliance, and set a tone for the treatment phase that emphasizes collaboration.

## HANDLING THE INITIAL CONTACT: CONDUCTING A BRIEF PHONE SCREEN

Today referrals can arrive from a variety of channels, including self-referrals from Internet listings or websites, colleagues, word of mouth, and insurance agencies. As a result, it is often beneficial to conduct a brief phone screen with the patient prior to scheduling an initial appointment. Along with using the phone screen to determine the chief complaint, a match for your clinical competencies, and eligibility for your practice, it may be wise to remember that from the moment initial contact is made, the patient's expectations for the treatment can be shaped and motivation for change enhanced.

For example, the initial phone screen may include an assessment of the patient's (1) current symptoms, (2) estimate of their severity, (3) previous treatment history, (4) understanding of CBT, (5) motivation and readiness to try CBT, and (6) current risk factors (e.g., drugs, alcohol, current suicidal ideation, homicidal ideation) or (7) other factors that may negatively impact treatment (e.g., nonsupportive family, time constraints, distance to office). In addition, the initial phone screen may be used to provide a brief overview of a typical course of treatment (e.g., assessment phase, treatment phase, approximate number of sessions), correct any misconceptions about CBT, and describe your available office hours, fee policies, and the like. Finally, as some patients experience considerable shame and fear about describing the content of their obsessions and/or the nature of their compulsions, the initial phone screen can be used to instill hope by normalizing symptoms (especially if this is the first time the patient will be entering into therapy) and providing general information on the treatment outcome data (as has been described earlier in this book). A sample Phone Screen Template can be found in Appendix B (Form 1).

If after the phone screen you determine that the patient is a good match for the services you offer (e.g., the patient's chief complaint matches your clinical competencies; your schedule matches, fees/health insurance are not an issue), you should set up a date and time for an intake evaluation (structured diagnostic interview and general clinical evaluation). As indicated on the sample Phone Screen Template (see Appendix B, Form 1), it can be useful to make sure the patient has the correct address for your office, as well as specific directions on how to find it. In addition, it can be helpful to provide information on how long the first session will be, whether significant others are wanted or allowed in the session, and any other supplemental information you would like the patient to bring in to the first session (e.g., a list of current and past medications, previous treatment providers, payment methods accepted). While somewhat of a heavy initial time investment, exchanging all of this information can help to ensure a smooth initial appointment.

Not all of the patients you screen will end up being suitable candidates for treatment with you. It is a normal and important aspect of professional identity development (as well as an ethical requirement) to be aware of the limits of your competencies. If a patient is not a suitable candidate for treatment with you (e.g., she presents with significant comorbid substance abuse issues, which you have not been trained to treat), it can be helpful to provide the patient with an explanation for why you are not setting up an appointment with her (e.g., outside of your area of competency or age ranges treated, incompatible schedules, not on their insurance panel). You should also have some additional resources or recommendations available for the patient, such as a colleague you can recommend with a clinical practice in her area who is accepting new referrals or a website that contains a listing of treatment providers in her area (see Appendix A for a list of helpful websites for finding a therapist).

## CONDUCTING AN INTAKE EVALUATION

As mentioned earlier, it is imperative that you always conduct a full and thorough intake evaluation to create a detailed, albeit preliminary, case formulation. That is, before beginning a course of CBT for OCD, it is imperative to gather enough information to (1) be confident that OCD is, in fact, the primary diagnosis; (2) account for biological, psychological (cognitions, emotions, and behaviors), and social factors involved the etiology and maintenance of the disorder; (3) understand the role of various mitigating and aggravating factors over the course of the disorder; and (4) assess for other factors that may complicate treatment (e.g., comorbid psychopathology, psychosocial stressors, medical conditions). As such, the intake evaluation should include a formal diagnostic assessment to screen for the presence of OCD as well as other psychiatric disorders and/ or symptoms (covered below) along with a more general clinical evaluation that reviews other biopsychosocial factors that may be impacting the patient and could exert an influence on treatment outcome (see Chapter 5). Although each of these two phases is described separately, they can be combined in any way the clinician deems appropriate (e.g., one longer session) and/or reversed in order of administration.

## STRUCTURED DIAGNOSTIC INTERVIEWS

Structured diagnostic interviews are useful for determining and verifying the primary diagnosis, assessing for comorbid diagnoses, and noting additional subthreshold symptoms. Currently, there are a number of empirically based structured diagnostic assessment tools to choose from, including (1) the Structured Clinical Interview for DSM Disorders (SCID), (2) the Anxiety Disorders Interview Schedule for DSM (ADIS), and (3) the Mini-International Neuropsychiatric Interview (MINI).

### Structured Clinical Interview for DSM Disorders

The SCID is a semistructured interview for making the major DSM diagnoses. (There is also a SCID-5-PD for making Personality Disorder diagnoses.) Several different versions are available, including a Research Version and a Clinician Version. The administration time of the SCID can vary greatly, depending on the extent of the patient's psychopathology and psychiatric history. It is estimated to range from about 15 minutes (i.e., a subject with virtually no psychopathology or psychiatric history) up to several hours (i.e., a subject with extensive psychiatric comorbidity, a long psychiatric history, and with a tangential and/or circumstantial style of speech). The average administration time of the full Research Version of the SCID is estimated at 90 minutes, and the average administration time for the SCID-5-PD is estimated at 45 minutes. All versions of the SCID, along with training tapes, interview guides, and response booklets, are copyrighted and must be purchased through American Psychiatric Publishing, Inc.

### Anxiety Disorders Interview Schedule for DSM

The ADIS is a structured interview designed to assess for current episodes of anxiety disorders in order to permit the differential diagnosis among the anxiety disorders according to DSM criteria, as well as provide sufficient information to permit a functional analysis of the anxiety disorders to be performed. It also includes modules that assess for current mood, somatoform, and substance use disorders—owing to their high comorbidity rate with the anxiety disorders and also to the fact that the presenting symptomatology of these disorders is often quite similar to that of the anxiety disorders. In addition, the ADIS contains screening questions for psychotic and conversion symptoms and familial psychiatric history, as well as a more detailed section to ascertain the patient's medical and psychiatric treatment history.

The ADIS, like the SCID, is also currently available in several different forms, including an Adult Version (ADIS-5) and a Lifetime Version (ADIS-5L). The Lifetime Version contains all of the sections included in the regular ADIS, while also being designed to establish past (lifetime) diagnoses and containing a diagnostic timeline to assist in determining the onset, remission, and temporal sequence of current and past disorders. The average administration time of the ADIS is estimated at 90 minutes, but some studies have reported much longer times, depending on the population and the extent of the patient's psychopathology and psychiatric history. It is suggested that clinicians administering the ADIS be trained in how to conduct the interview, and a clinician's manual has been developed for both the regular ADIS and the Lifetime Version. All versions are available from Oxford University Press.

## Mini–International Neuropsychiatric Interview

The MINI is a short, structured diagnostic interview that was developed in 1990 by psychiatrists and clinicians in the United States and Europe for DSM-IV and ICD-10 psychiatric disorders. According to its publishers, it is the most widely used psychiatric structured diagnostic interview instrument in the world and is currently employed by mental health professionals and health organizations in more than 100 countries. Although the standard MINI does not provide the same level of detail as the SCID or ADIS, it is much briefer (estimated administration time of the standard MINI is approximately 15 minutes) and has been validated against the SCID, as well as against the Composite International Diagnostic Interview for ICD-10 (CIDI)—and even against expert opinion in a large sample in four European countries (France, the United Kingdom, Italy, and Spain). As such, many researchers consider it to be a fully validated and more time-efficient alternative to the SCID and ADIS.

Like the SCID and ADIS, the MINI is currently available in several different forms, all of which are bundled into a "MINI Suite" by the publisher. The suite includes the regular MINI (in different languages such as Cantonese, English, Finnish, German, Gujarati, Hindi, Japanese, Korean, Latvian, Malay, Mandarin Chinese for Taiwan, Polish, Romanian, Russian, Serbian, Spanish for the United States, Swedish, Tagalog, Telugu, Ukraine); the MINI "Plus" (which is more comprehensive in disorders assessed); the MINI for ADHD Studies; the MINI for Schizophrenia and Psychotic Disorders Studies; the MINI "Kid" (in different languages such as Austrian German, Bulgarian, Cebuano, Croatian, Dutch for Belgium, Dutch for the Netherlands, English, Estonian, Finish, French for Belgium, Gujarati, Greek, Hungarian, Italian, Korean, Lithuanian, Malay for Malaysia, Malay for Singapore, Malayalam, Mandarin Chinese for Malaysia, Marathi, Polish, Romanian, Russian for Estonia, Russian for Lithuania, Simplified Chinese for Singapore, Spanish for the US, Swedish for Sweden, Tagalog); the MINI "Kid" for Schizophrenia and Psychotic Disorders Studies; and a MINI Screening tool. The "MINI Suite" is available from Medical Outcome Systems, Inc. It currently comes in several different forms and has different costs, depending on whether it is to be used by students or organizations and on whether interviews will be done manually, through the web, or on a desktop computer.

# DIFFERENTIAL DIAGNOSIS

Although the structured diagnostic interviews described above will assist in the accurate screening and diagnosis of patients, it should be noted that (1) patients typically present with comorbid psychopathology—be it in the form of additional diagnoses or subthreshold clusters of symptoms, and, perhaps as a result of this; (2) a trend has been emerging in treatment outcome studies in which there has been a shift away from diagnostically driven interventions toward interventions targeting the cognitive and behavioral *mechanisms* hypothesized to underlie various disorders. A full discussion of the latter is beyond the scope of this chapter (see Barlow, Allen, & Choate, 2004), but an exploration of the former, as it applies to accurately differentially diagnosing OCD, is warranted at this time.

Differentially diagnosing OCD from other disorders can be a challenge for a number of reasons, including: (1) OCD is known to co-occur with other disorders at a high rate, (2) a number of other disorders have symptoms that are similar to OCD, and (3) as previously mentioned, the terms *obsession* and *compulsion* have now been incorporated into our daily language. Currently, most DSM diagnostic criteria contain the instruction to give a specific diagnosis only if the symptoms are not better accounted for by another disorder. Attributing a symptom to OCD instead of another disorder, however, is not always an easy task. Fortunately, much has been written on the proposed differences between OCD and other disorders, which can be useful for clinicians to consider when they are attempting to make a differential diagnosis. A review of some of the key disorders that have similar presenting complaints is presented next and is followed by a summary chart (Figure 4.1) for aiding in the differential diagnosis of OCD.

## Generalized Anxiety Disorder

Patients with generalized anxiety disorder also present with significant anxiety and excessive worries that can often resemble the obsessions found in OCD. One way to differentiate the two is to observe that patients with generalized anxiety disorder usually report that their fears are more reality-based (e.g., about financial stresses, academic or work performance, or the health of an aging loved one) than the content found in typical obsessions. In addition, the worries of patients with generalized anxiety disorder tend to be less bizarre than the obsessive thoughts of patients with OCD, and their worry themes may shift more frequently over time, while there appears to be more of a stability in the content of obsessions.

## Panic Disorder

Although panic attacks are the central symptom in panic disorder, they also commonly occur across the anxiety disorders, including OCD. One way to differentiate panic disorder from OCD is that patients with panic disorder must experience at least some attacks that are unexpected or uncued, and they are primarily anxious about experiencing another attack and the consequences of the attack. In contrast, patients with OCD typically will experience panic attacks only when confronting their OCD triggers and will not typically worry about the consequence of the attacks per se, but rather the consequence related to their OCD theme.

| Is the patient . . . | Then the diagnosis is more likely . . . |
|---|---|
| Preoccupied with unwanted intrusive thoughts that are more reality-based, worries that are less bizarre, and worry themes that shift frequently over time? | Generalized anxiety disorder |
| Experiencing panic attacks, at least some of which occur unexpectedly/without any trigger, with the fear primarily centering on experiencing another attack and/or the consequences of the attack? | Panic disorder |
| Preoccupied with unwanted intrusive thoughts that tend to be exclusively related to situations in which he or she may be judged negatively or do something to embarrass him- or herself and yet is able to effectively use avoidance in order to manage his or her obsessive thoughts? | Social anxiety disorder |
| Preoccupied with unwanted intrusive thoughts and rituals that are invariably connected to a past traumatic event? | Posttraumatic stress disorder |
| Preoccupied with unwanted and repetitive negative thoughts that are oriented more toward the past than future, are more general thoughts about the patient's failures and misgivings, feel more volitional and reality-based in nature, are not actively resisted, frequently shift in theme over time, and lead to more of a depressed mood than anxious mood? | Major depressive disorder |
| Preoccupied with unwanted intrusive thoughts that are invariably connected to concerns about his or her health and/or a preoccupation with bodily symptoms and/or sensations? | Somatic symptom disorder or illness anxiety disorder |
| Preoccupied with unwanted intrusive thoughts that are invariably connected to concerns about an imagined defect in appearance or an exaggerated sense of the severity of a perceived physical flaw? | Body dysmorphic disorder |
| Preoccupied with compulsive and repetitive pulling behaviors that are at times performed outside of awareness (i.e., in the absence of obsessive thoughts or a "need" to ritualize) and/or at times experienced as appetitive? | Trichotillomania |
| Preoccupied with compulsive and repetitive skin picking that is at times performed outside of awareness (i.e., in the absence of obsessive thoughts or a "need" to ritualize) and/or at times experienced as appetitive? | Excoriation (skin-picking) disorder |
| Preoccupied with repetitive movements and acts that serve to reduce sensory tension (premonitory urges) rather than manage feelings of anxiety generated by obsessive thoughts? | Tourette's disorder |

(*continued*)

**FIGURE 4.1.** Chart for aiding in the differential diagnosis of OCD.

| Is the patient . . . | Then the diagnosis is more likely . . . |
|---|---|
| Preoccupied with unwanted intrusive thoughts that are invariably connected to concerns about food, body image, weight, and eating and/or engaged in compulsions that focus on diet, exercise, eating, and food preparation that are at times experienced as appetitive only resisted because of their deleterious consequences? | Anorexia nervosa, bulimia nervosa, or binge-eating disorder |
| A perfectionist, with fixed, rigid notions and expectations about how daily activities should be performed and relationships should be managed; considered to be difficult and stubborn; viewed by others as cold and indifferent; not bothered by these traits and in fact, sees them as functional and adaptive, and therefore does not try to resist them? | Obsessive–compulsive personality disorder |
| Preoccupied with unwanted intrusive thoughts that are invariably connected to concerns about something important being discarded by accident that will have a potential value or use or some sentimental meaning such that the patient has persistent difficulty getting rid of his or her possessions, to the point that the amount of clutter disrupts his or her ability to use his or her living or work spaces—and yet does not cause distress, so urges to collect and hoard are rarely resisted? | Hoarding disorder |
| Preoccupied with unwanted intrusive thoughts that are invariably connected to concerns that his or her body is emitting a foul and unpleasant odor that may offend others? | Olfactory reference syndrome |

**FIGURE 4.1**   (*continued*)

## Social Anxiety Disorder

Whereas patients with social anxiety disorder and those with OCD may worry about offending others, patients with social anxiety disorder tend to be concerned exclusively about situations in which they may be judged negatively or do something to embarrass themselves, and patients with OCD tend to have more varied concerns. In addition, whereas patients with OCD can never entirely avoid their obsessions, patients with social anxiety disorder are often able to use avoidance to manage their fears.

## Posttraumatic Stress Disorder

Patients diagnosed with PTSD also report experiencing recurrent, intrusive thoughts and/or engaging in rituals, but with PTSD, the unwanted intrusive thoughts and rituals are invariably connected to a past traumatic event. For example, a victim of a sexual assault may experience unwanted intrusive thoughts about the sexual assault and/or engage in washing rituals (repeated showers or baths) and checking rituals (door locks, windows, etc.) to feel safe after the traumatic event.

## Major Depressive Disorder

Patients diagnosed with major depressive disorder also report experiencing repetitive negative thoughts, which are often termed "ruminations" as opposed to obsessions. Some researchers suggest that ruminations differ from obsessions and worries in that they tend to be oriented more toward the past than the future, are more general thoughts about the patient, her life, and her future, and are often either more volitional in nature, or at least not resisted as strongly or seen as unrealistic. In addition, as was the case of worries in patients with generalized anxiety disorder, the theme of the ruminations may shift frequently over time, while there appears to be more of stability in the content of obsessions.

## OCD "Spectrum" Disorders

As mentioned earlier, a number of other disorders have strikingly similar symptom patterns to OCD. In addition, their course, comorbidity, biological abnormalities, and treatment responses all appear similar to those in OCD. As a result, these disorders are frequently described in the literature as obsessive–compulsive "spectrum" disorders. As mentioned in Chapter 1 and highlighted below, some of these disorders have now been grouped with OCD in a new chapter in the DSM-5 called "Obsessive–Compulsive and Related Disorders." Following is a brief summary of these disorders.

## Hypochondriasis

Hypochondriasis, previously classified as a somatoform disorder, was eliminated as a disorder in DSM-5. Many of the patients who would have previously been diagnosed with hypochondriasis are now likely to receive the DSM-5 diagnosis of somatic symptom disorder (i.e., a patient who has significant somatic symptoms as well as a high level of health anxiety). If, however, the patient has a high level of health anxiety *without somatic symptoms*, then he will likely receive a DSM-5 diagnosis of illness anxiety disorder (unless his health anxiety is better explained by a primary anxiety disorder, such as generalized anxiety disorder). Compared to OCD, however, in somatic symptom disorder, the recurrent ideas about somatic symptoms or illness are typically experienced as less intrusive and, perhaps as a result, patients with somatic symptom disorder also do not typically engage in the associated rituals for reducing anxiety that occur in patients with OCD. Patients with illness anxiety disorder may report experiencing intrusive thoughts about having a disease and engaging in associated rituals for reducing anxiety (e.g., seeking reassurance). In illness anxiety disorder, the preoccupations are usually focused on *having a disease*, whereas in OCD, the thoughts are usually focused on fears of *getting a disease* in the future. Moreover, most patients with OCD also report experiencing obsessions or compulsions involving other concerns in addition to their fears about contracting a disease.

## Body Dysmorphic Disorder

Historically classified as a somatoform disorder, in DSM-5 body dysmorphic disorder is grouped together with OCD in a new, separate chapter called "Obsessive–Compulsive and Related Disorders." Body dysmorphic disorder involves an obsessive, irrational preoccupation with a real or an imagined defect in physical appearance. If a slight physical anomaly is present, the person's concern is markedly excessive and cannot be better accounted for by another mental disorder (e.g., dissatisfaction with body shape and size in anorexia nervosa). In both body dysmorphic disorder and OCD, repetitive behaviors or mental acts in response to preoccupations with perceived defects or flaws in physical appearance may be observed. However, people with OCD tend to have other obsessions and compulsions, whereas the concerns in body dysmorphic disorder are limited to one's physical appearance.

## Trichotillomania

Historically classified as an impulse-control disorder, in DSM-5 "hair-pulling disorder" was added parenthetically to this disorder's name, and it is grouped together with OCD in a new, separate chapter called "Obsessive–Compulsive and Related Disorders." Trichotillomania (hair-pulling disorder) involves the recurrent failure to resist impulses to pull out one's own hair, from any region on the body in which hair grows, resulting in hair loss. Previously, in order to meet the criteria for this disorder, the patient needed to experience an increasing sense of tension immediately before pulling out the hair or when attempting to resist the behavior, along with pleasure, relief, or gratification from the hair pulling. More recent data, however, suggest that some patients do not experience the rising tension followed by relief, this criterion was dropped in DSM-5. Trichotillomania can be differentiated from OCD by the fact that in trichotillomania, the compulsive behavior is limited to hair pulling and is performed in the absence of obsessions.

## Compulsive Skin Picking

As is the case of trichotillomania, compulsive skin picking (also previously referred to as dermatillomania and neurotic excoriation) has historically been classified as an impulse-control disorder. In DSM-5, however, it was renamed excoriation (skin-picking) disorder and grouped together with OCD, body dysmorphic disorder, and trichotillomania in a new, separate chapter called "Obsessive–Compulsive and Related Disorders." Excoriation disorder involves the repetitive picking at one's own skin so that the skin becomes noticeably damaged. Although the most common locations are usually the face, arms, and hands, the picking can be directed at any part of the body. The picking may target healthy skin, normal skin variations (e.g., freckles and moles), preexisting blemishes (e.g., scabs, sores, or acne), or imagined skin defects that nobody else can observe. Also, as is the case with trichotillomania, the compulsive behavior is limited to skin picking in the absence of obsessions, which does not fit with the diagnosis of OCD.

## Tourette's Disorder

Technically classified as a tic disorder, Tourette's disorder involves both multiple motor (e.g., eye blink, nose twitch, grimace) and one or more vocal (e.g., including grunting, throat clearing, shouting, swearing) tics that appear in early childhood or adolescence (before the age of 18 years), seem to occur for no reason, and last for more than one year. Studies have found high rates of

OCD symptoms in Tourette's disorder sufferers (with some studies showing rates as high as 74%) and high rates of Tourette's disorder symptoms in OCD sufferers (with some studies showing rates as high as 35%). As a result, DSM-5 notes that differentiating obsessive–compulsive behaviors from tics may be difficult. Many persons with Tourette's disorder, however, report what are described as premonitory urges (the urge to perform a motor activity), with the touching, repetitive movements and acts that look like compulsions actually serving to reduce sensory tension rather than manage feelings of anxiety generated by obsessions. Clues favoring OCD include a more cognitive-based trigger (e.g., fear of contamination) and/or a need to perform the action in a particular fashion a certain number of times, equally on both sides of the body, or until a "just right" feeling is achieved.

## Eating Disorders (Anorexia Nervosa, Bulimia Nervosa, and Binge–Eating Disorder)

Anorexia nervosa involves the failure to maintain a healthy, normal body weight through restriction of eating or eating followed by purging. Bulimia nervosa involves binge eating with a feeling of no control during binge-eating episodes, followed by compensation through fasting, purging, or extreme exercise to prevent weight gain. Binge-eating disorder involves recurrent episodes of binge eating in the absence of regular use of compensatory behaviors characteristic of bulimia nervosa. Studies have found high rates of OCD symptoms in patients with eating disorders (with some studies showing symptom rates as high as 88%), as well as high rates of eating disorders in patients diagnosed with OCD. In addition, individuals suffering from eating disorders may experience obsessive thoughts about food, body image, weight, and eating, and may also appear to engage in compulsions surrounding diet, exercise, eating, and food preparation. As is the case with the impulse-control disorders, however, these activities are not generally considered to be compulsions as defined by the DSM because the person usually finds them appetitive and may wish to resist them only because of their deleterious consequences—neither of which function fits with the diagnosis of OCD. In addition, in OCD the obsessions and compulsions are typically not limited to concerns about weight and food.

## Other Possible Obsessive- and Compulsive-Like Behaviors

Other obsessive- and compulsive-like behaviors that are important to consider when making a differential diagnosis include (1) olfactory reference syndrome, the obsessive, irrational fear that one's body is emitting a foul and unpleasant odor that may offend others; (2) compulsive sexual behavior, a broad category that is generally divided into two subcategories: paraphilic or irregular sexual behaviors (e.g., pedophilia, voyeurism, exhibitionism, frotteurism) and nonparaphilic or normal sexual behaviors taken to levels so extreme they cause extreme distress and impairment; (3) gambling disorder (characterized by an "obsessive" need to gamble, which leads to clinically significant impairment or distress); and (4) various other impulse-control disorders, such as intermittent explosive disorder (characterized by episodes of uncontrollable rage and anger), pyromania (intentionally setting a fire for gratification), and kleptomania (characterized by the impulsive need to steal). Although many of these disorders include behaviors that are sometimes described as "compulsive," these behaviors differ from the compulsions of OCD in that the person usually derives pleasure from the activity and may wish to resist it only because of its deleterious consequences.

## Obsessive–Compulsive Personality Disorder

Whereas OCD and obsessive–compulsive personality disorder share similar names, they are very different disorders. For example, in contrast to OCD, patients with Obsessive-Compulsive Personality Disorder rarely report experiencing intense obsessions and engaging in as frequent compulsions as those with OCD. Instead, patients with obsessive–compulsive personality disorder tend to be perfectionists, with fixed, rigid notions and expectations about how daily activities should be performed and relationships should be managed. As a result, they are often considered to be difficult and stubborn, as they tend to see their way of doing things as the only way. They can also be seen as cold and indifferent, as they sometimes struggle to express warm and loving emotions. People with obsessive–compulsive personality disorder, however, tend to view their traits as functional and adaptive, and therefore do not find their symptoms to be upsetting and do not try to resist them.

## A Special Note on Hoarding

Hoarding shares many similarities with OCD, such as obsessive fears that something important might be discarded by accident (e.g., a passport may have ended up in a section of the newspaper), that something may have a potential value or use (which is distinguished from hobbies and/or collecting objects of monetary value), or that an object could have some sentimental meaning (e.g., memory of a person). Though not as common, hoarding can also include the obsessive fear of losing something symbolic to the person, such as part of their "essence" when they get up from a chair. In addition, in response to these obsessive fears, hoarding involves collecting compulsions, such as buying a large number of items on sale, saving items for a later use, or being unwilling to discard seemingly useless items. Though not as common, hoarding can also include retrieving useless items from the trash, hoarding animals, and hoarding bodily waste and fluids.

Perhaps as a result of these similarities, hoarding has traditionally been considered a symptom of OCD and has historically been included in most structured clinical interviews and measures of OCD symptoms. There are differences, however, that have led to a continuing debate about whether hoarding should be seen as a separate disorder. For example, for many patients who hoard, the hoarding does not cause distress and therefore urges to collect and hoard are rarely resisted. On the contrary, many patients who hoard generally believe that the collection and retention of objects is desirable and perhaps even necessary, even if perhaps slightly out of hand. In addition, hoarding is also listed as a symptom of several other disorders, including schizophrenia and eating disorders; in brain-injured patients, hoarding accompanied by self-neglect and living in squalor is also considered to be a symptom of Diogenes syndrome, which is found in some older individuals.

Hoarding is not directly mentioned in the DSM as a symptom of OCD. Rather, a description most closely matching that of hoarding ("the inability to discard worn-out or worthless objects even when they have no sentimental value") has traditionally been found as one of the criteria of obsessive–compulsive personality disorder. Only when describing the differential diagnosis between obsessive–compulsive personality disorder and OCD has the DSM made any explicit link between OCD and hoarding. For example, the DSM-IV-TR stated:

> Despite the similarity in names, OCD is usually easily distinguished from Obsessive–Compulsive Personality Disorder by the presence of true obsessions and compulsions. A diagnosis of OCD should be considered especially when hoarding is extreme (e.g. accumulated stacks of worthless objects present a fire hazard and make it difficult for others to walk through the house). (American Psychiatric Association, 2000, p. 728)

Thus, though not explicitly stated in the OCD section of the DSM, it has been assumed that, when severe, hoarding could be considered a symptom of OCD.

As mentioned earlier, in DSM-5 (American Psychiatric Association, 2013), hoarding has become an official diagnosis onto itself ("hoarding disorder") and is grouped with OCD in a new, separate chapter called "Obsessive–Compulsive and Related Disorders" as both a reflection of more recent evidence of the interrelatedness of these disorders and the clinical utility of grouping them together in the same chapter. An excellent paper by Mataix-Cols et al. (2010) provides a focused review of the literature on hoarding and presents a number of options and recommendations that ultimately were adopted in DSM-5.

## COMORBID CONDITIONS

Even after conducting a thorough differential diagnosis of other disorders with symptoms that are similar to OCD, it is still likely that additional, comorbid conditions will be diagnosed along with the OCD, as it is known to co-occur with other disorders at a high rate. These can include other anxiety disorders (e.g., generalized anxiety disorder, social anxiety disorder, panic disorder, separation anxiety disorder) and mood disorders (e.g., major depressive disorder and bipolar disorder), as well as attention-deficit/hyperactivity disorder, tic disorders, trichotillomania, body dysmorphic disorder, and somatoform disorders. The most commonly diagnosed comorbid conditions appear to be depressive disorders (affecting more than one-half of the subjects in some studies) and other anxiety disorders (affecting more than one-quarter of the subjects in some studies).

Of the anxiety disorders, panic disorder, and generalized anxiety disorder have been the two most commonly found to co-occur with OCD. Of note has been the consistent finding of personality disorders in individuals diagnosed with OCD—although prevalence rates have varied widely (approximately between 5 and 30%, but can be much higher, depending on how the subjects were assessed). Of the personality disorders, avoidant, dependent, histrionic, schizotypal, and obsessive–compulsive personality disorder are the most frequently diagnosed along with OCD.

The extent and type of comorbidity between OCD and other disorders appear to be somewhat age-related. For example, adolescents with OCD seem to suffer from a significantly higher rate of major depressive disorder than do children with OCD, while children with OCD seem to suffer from a significantly higher rate of separation anxiety disorder than do adolescents with OCD.

## TAKE-HOME MESSAGE

With the creation and dissemination of evidence-based treatment protocols, it is easy for clinicians to perform a quick, superficial assessment and then dive into treatment without conducting a careful and detailed assessment of the patient's presenting problem(s). And while cognitive-behavioral therapies (including Ex/RP) are often robust enough to help many patients treated in this superficial manner, it will be of greater benefit in the more complex or severe cases to take the time (usually one or two sessions) to conduct a thorough initial evaluation in order to create a preliminary case formulation (see Chapter 5) that will prepare the patient for treatment and to maximize the potential for a positive treatment outcome. The first steps include (1) conducting a brief phone screen and (2) completing a formal diagnostic assessment to screen for the presence of OCD as well as other psychiatric disorders and/or symptoms. This can then be combined with a more general clinical evaluation that reviews other biopsychosocial factors that may be impacting the patient and could exert an influence on treatment outcome, as well as evidence-based, clinician-administered OCD-specific assessment measures and other evidence-based self-report measures (see Chapter 5). Although each of these two phases is described separately, they can in fact be combined in any way the clinician deems appropriate (e.g., one longer session and/or reversed in order of administration).

# Clinical Evaluation
# and Case Formulation

Along with a *structured diagnostic evaluation* (see Chapter 4), it is important to place the patient's presenting symptoms in the context of both his or her current living environment and life history. Conducting a *general clinical evaluation* will help flesh out these issues and, in so doing, generate information that can be combined with the information obtained from the structured diagnostic evaluation, as well as any evidence-based *clinician-administered* OCD-specific assessment measures and/or evidence-based *self-report* measures, in order to create a comprehensive biopsychosocial *case formulation*.

## ELEMENTS OF A GENERAL CLINICAL EVALUATION

The general clinical evaluation should include information on the following areas.

### Identifying Information

Obtain the patient's name, date of birth, age, gender, ethnicity, marital status, children, living status, financial status, and referral source.

### Chief Complaint or Presenting Problems

Using the patient's words, generate a list of problem areas and/or symptoms (focusing on affective, cognitive, behavioral symptoms, as well as symptom severity). It is also important to gather OCD-specific information. This should include (1) external triggers (i.e., objects or situations that make the patient anxious), such as touching door handles, locking a door, doing laundry; (2) internal triggers (i.e., thoughts, images, impulses or body sensations that make the patient anxious), such as images of loved ones dying in an accident, thoughts about certain numbers, and beliefs about being contaminated, as well as tingling or numbness, aches and pains, racing heart, and swallowing; (3) preliminary appraisals of the thoughts; (4) feared consequences of external and internal triggers (e.g., contracting AIDS after touching a brown spot on the wall); (5) rituals performed, including both observable behaviors and mental rituals; (6) any situations or triggers that the patient avoids either actively (e.g., not shaking hands, not using public bathrooms) or passively (e.g., allowing someone else to open a bathroom door in order to leave the bathroom without touching the doorknob); and (7) any "safety behaviors" that the patient engages in to help manage difficult situations. Often, these are not as obvious as rituals and/or may seem more normative. These include using antibacterial lotions to "decontaminate" one's hands, using a paper towel to turn off sink faucets or open a bathroom door, and flushing a toilet with one's foot.

## History of the Presenting Illness

Given that much of the information obtained up to this point will have been in the present or here-and-now, it can also be useful to collect information about the history of the patient's OCD. This history should include when the patient first recalls experiencing the symptoms of OCD, along with any remarkable circumstances that were taking place around the time symptoms began. Once details about the onset have been documented, the clinician should then focus on precipitating factors, maintaining factors, and any cycling of symptoms, and note times/factors associated with improvements and deteriorations. If this is done following the use of a structured diagnostic instrument (e.g., MINI), you should focus on the OCD but include any other disorders diagnosed during that portion of the interview. If you are not using a structured diagnostic instrument (or if you are doing the general intake evaluation first), you should focus on the chief complaint and return for more history as additional problem areas/diagnoses are identified—including potential functional connections between the different problem areas.

## Psychiatric Treatment History

Obtain information on any inpatient treatment (including reason, dates, length of stay, diagnosis and treatments, response to treatment); outpatient treatment (including reason, dates, length of treatment, session frequency, provider's approach); and substance abuse treatment (including reason, dates, length of stay, diagnosis and treatments, response to treatment). It may also be useful to have the patient complete a Release of Information form for any key providers. In addition, it is important to inquire about any history of suicidal ideation or attempts, as well as any current suicidal ideation (if not already discussed earlier in the evaluation). Similarly, but often neglected, is the importance of inquiring about any history of violence or assaults, any current or past homicidal ideation, or issues that may impact the patient's dangerousness. Finally, you should ask whether the patient has engaged in any nonsuicidal self-injurious behaviors (e.g., cutting, biting, scratching), in the past or more recently.

## Medical History

Measure (or ask for) the patient's height and weight and use these data to calculate a body mass index (BMI).[1] Inquire about the patient's current and past medical problems/illnesses/diseases.

---

[1]There are numerous free online services (e.g., the National Institutes of Health or the Centers for Disease Control and Prevention) and apps that can help calculate the BMI.

Encourage the patient to have a full physical examination if one has not been performed in the past year and get written permission to discuss the findings with the patient's physician, as most psychiatric diagnoses are given only if the symptoms are not due to the direct physiological effects of a general medical condition. It can also be useful to obtain information on the patient's lifestyle, in terms of both nutrition (e.g., well nourished/fed, obesity/emaciation, recent weight gain/loss, increased appetite, bingeing) and exercise (e.g., how active, how much working out).

## Medication History

If the patient brought in a list of current and past medications, take a few moments to review it with him during the session. If the patient was not instructed to bring in a list during the initial phone contact (see Chapter 4) or forgot to bring it in, it is useful to record some basic information and then ask him to bring the list to the next session. Be sure that the list includes the names of both current and past psychiatric and nonpsychiatric medications, along with the dose, the reason for taking them, how the medications were prescribed, whether the patient is taking them as prescribed, if the patient has had any positive response to them, whether the patient experienced any side effects, and if, discontinued, the reason for stopping. Obtain written permission to discuss the findings with the patient's psychiatrist/prescriber. It is also useful to get information on any nonpsychiatric medications the patient is taking (e.g., herbals, vitamins) and any allergies the patient has to medications.

## Alcohol and Substance Use History

If not covered during the structured diagnostic evaluation (see Chapter 4), it is important to obtain information on the patient's use of alcohol and other substances, including nicotine, caffeine, and prescription medications (used at doses higher or for purposes other than prescribed). Obtain information on when the patient first started using, the period of heaviest use, the last time used, current average use, the relation of use (if any) to the patient's symptoms, and the overall impact that drugs and alcohol have had on the patient's life.

## Family History

It is important to take into account the patient's family history of psychiatric, medical, and substance abuse issues, as this history may shed light on both biological and psychological vulnerabilities the patient may have "inherited"—genetically and/or through social learning. Obtain information on each, including the nature of the family member's relationship to the patient (e.g., mother, paternal aunt, paternal first cousin), diagnosis, treatments, and current status. Pay attention to both biological/genetic risk factors and psychological risk factors such as cognitive biases that may have been learned through information provision, direct experience, or role modeling. It is also useful to obtain the current status of the patient's parents and/or siblings (e.g., alive or deceased, location, frequency of contact, nature of relationship). Finally, given the current prevalence estimates, if not covered during the structured diagnostic evaluation (see Chapter 4), it is important to inquire about any history of abuse or traumas in the patient's life, including sexual, physical, or emotional abuse or neglect.

## Personal/Social History

It is also important to account for the role that social, cultural, and other environmental factors may have played or continue to play in the course of the disorder. As such, getting a detailed personal history is crucial and should include (1) where the patient was born and raised and any significant events during childhood that may be connected to the chief complaint; (2) an academic/educational history, with highest level achieved, performance in school, and any education-related issues resulting from, or contributing to, the patient's symptoms; (3) the patient's current work status (e.g., satisfaction from job, stress level at work, relationship satisfaction with coworkers, boss) and employment history, including any work-related issues as a result of, or contributing to, the patient's symptoms; (4) a history of significant relationships, both romantic and friendships, including size of, and satisfaction with, current social network, whether any people in it are aware of the patient's disorder, and if the patient can confide/seek support from anyone; and (5) a legal history, including charges, arrests, and convictions.

## Mental Status Examination

The mental status examination provides a comprehensive and structured description of the patient's current mental state. Numerous forms and checklists are available online[2] for free that can assist in conducting a mental status examination, with most including the domains of appearance, general behavior, attitude toward the examiner, state of consciousness, attention, orientation, psychomotor activity, mood, affect, speech, form of thought, content of thought, perceptions, insight, memory, judgment, and intellectual functioning.

## Preliminary DSM Diagnosis

Though not critical to include, in certain settings (e.g., academic medical centers) it can be useful to summarize all of the diagnostic information obtained into a preliminary assessment. Information on how to do this can be found in the first section of DSM-5 ("Use of the Manual"). Having a summary of the diagnoses, including a note about which are primary and which (if any) are provisional and/or subthreshold can allow you (and others who may be sharing care of the case in a medical setting) to quickly focus on the main areas of concern and main symptoms being targeted in treatment.

## Augmenting the Evaluation with Evidence-Based, Clinician-Administered OCD-Specific Assessment Measures

After using a structured diagnostic interview to confirm a (primary) diagnosis of OCD and then conducting a general clinical evaluation in order to determine the course of the disorder and place the diagnosis in the context of the patient's life, it is wise to augment the evaluation with one or more evidence-based clinician-administered tools for assessing various aspects of OCD. This can be done using structured assessment measures such as the Yale–Brown Obsessive–Compulsive

---

[2]Entering the key words "mental status exam form" into a search engine such as Google will produce over 1,630,000 results.

Scale (Y-BOCS; Goodman et al., 1989), the Brown Assessment of Beliefs Scale (BABS; Eisen, 1998), and the Overvalued Ideas Scale (OVIS; Neziroglu, McKay, Yaryura-Tobias, Stevens, & Todaro, 1999). The Y-BOCS is the gold-standard clinician-administered measure of OCD severity that has been used for decades in treatment outcomes studies, and the BABS and OVIS are scales that measure insight into the symptoms or disorder.

## Yale–Brown Obsessive–Compulsive Scale

The Y-BOCS (Goodman et al., 1989) consists of two forms. The first is a 64-item clinician-administered checklist that asks about the presence of various obsessions and compulsions, both currently and in the past. The checklist covers all of the major types of OCD symptoms (e.g., aggressive, contamination, sexual, religious, symmetry and exactness, somatic, as well as several miscellaneous symptoms). It also includes some symptoms of obsessive–compulsive spectrum disorders (trichotillomania, hoarding, hypochondriasis, etc.). After identifying all of the current symptoms, the most prominent symptoms are recorded on a target symptom list and then used as the basis for the second form, which is a 10-item clinician-administered semistructured interview that measures the severity of obsessions and compulsions. Each item is rated on a 5-point scale, ranging from 0 (no symptoms) to 4 (extremely severe symptoms), with respect to time spent, interference, distress, resistance, and control. These scores are combined to generate separate ratings of severity of obsessions (0–20) and compulsions (0–20), as well as an overall rating of severity of OCD (0–40).

The Y-BOCS takes about 30 minutes to administer but can take longer if the patient's OCD symptoms are numerous or particularly complex. A Y-BOCS score equal to or greater than 16 has historically been the cutoff score used to indicate clinically significant OCD in clinical trials. In addition, scores from 0 to 7 are considered to be indicative of subclinical OCD, with 8–15 representing mild OCD, 16–23 being considered moderate OCD, 24–31 severe, and 32–40 extreme. A more thorough description, along with a description of the original source, psychometric properties, alternative forms (e.g., the CYBOCS for children), and a reprint of the measure, are all available in *Practitioner's Guide to Empirically Based Measures of Anxiety* by Antony, Orsillo, and Roemer (2001), an excellent volume in the Association for Behavioral and Cognitive Therapies (ABCT) Clinical Assessment Series.

## Brown Assessment of Beliefs Scale

The BABS (Eisen, 1998) is a seven-item clinician-administered semistructured scale designed to assess the patient's degree of insight into the senselessness of the OCD symptoms (i.e., presence of delusional thinking). The BABS begins by having the therapist and patient determine one or two of the patient's dominant obsessional fears that have preoccupied the patient and/or been of significant concern during the previous week. It is important to note that the belief and associated consequences underlying it must be determined (e.g., that AIDS could be contracted by touching any object outside the home). Once this is completed, the clinician asks specific questions aimed at (1) assessing the patient's conviction as to validity of his fears, (2) examining his perceptions of how other people may view the validity of these fears, (3) if different, explaining why other people may hold a different view, (4) being willing to challenge his fears, (5) attempting to disprove the fears, (6) providing insight into whether his fears are a part of a psychological disorder, and (7) evaluating delusions of reference. Each question has five anchors, with descriptions corresponding to each anchor. The score for each item ranges from 0 (nondelusional/least pathological) to 4 (delusional/most pathological) and is meant to represent an average score for the past week. Only the first six items are included in the total score. More information on the scale and its psychometric properties is available in the original validation paper by Eisen et al. (1998).

## Overvalued Ideas Scale

The OVIS (Neziroglu et al., 1999) is a 10-item clinician-administered scale designed to measure the extent of a patient's strength of belief in the OCD symptoms. The OVIS begins with an open-ended question asking the patient to record the most prominent OCD-related belief that has been present in the past week. Once this is completed, the clinician asks nine questions that measure different aspects of the patient's belief: (1) strength, (2) reasonableness, (3) accuracy, (4) strength over past week, (5) extent to which others share the same belief, (6) how the patient attributes similar or differing beliefs, (7) how effective the patient's compulsions are, (8) the extent to which the disorder has caused the obsessive belief, and (9) the patient's degree of resistance to the belief. Each item is rated on a 10-point scale, ranging from 1 to 10, with the average of the items providing an estimate of overvalued ideation and higher scores representing greater levels of overvalued ideation. A more thorough description, along with a description of the original source, psychometric properties, alternative forms, and a reprint of the measure, are all available in Antony et al. (2001).

# ASSIGNING A COMPREHENSIVE EMPIRICALLY BASED SELF–REPORT MEASURES PACKET

In addition to all of the information gathered during the structured diagnostic interview and general clinical evaluation, it can be useful to have the patient complete a packet of empirically based self-report measures. This will allow for the objective and structured measurement of various aspects of OCD and comparisons to be made with established norms, while also normalizing symptoms and increasing the treatment's focus onto key target areas. The measures can also then be used as outcome measures (if administered at pre- and posttreatment, as well as at any follow-up or "booster" visits) and/or process measures (if administered at regularly spaced intervals throughout the treatment).

If using a comprehensive, empirically based packet of self-report measures, it would be wise to include (1) a cover sheet explaining the purpose of the packet, instructions on how to complete the measures, a rationale for their use in treatment, what to do if the patient has questions or concerns, and so on; (2) general information-gathering forms aimed at obtaining information on the person's personal and social history, a description of presenting problems, expectations regarding therapy, and the like (e.g., the Multimodal Life History Inventory [Lazarus & Lazarus, 1991], a 15-page data collection questionnaire divided into sections on general information, personal and social history, description of presenting problems, expectations regarding therapy, and a comprehensive modality analysis of current problems); (3) select self-report measures for OCD (e.g., the Obsessive–Compulsive Inventory—Revised, the Florida Obsessive–Compulsive Inventory, the Leyton Obsessional Inventory—Short Form, the Maudsley Obsessional–Compulsive Inventory, the Padua Inventory—Revised, the Obsessive Beliefs Questionnaire, the Interpretation of Intrusions Inventory, the Family Accommodation Scale); and (4) select self-report measures for commonly comorbid disorders, such as panic disorder and agoraphobia (e.g., the Panic Disorder Severity Scale—Self-Report), generalized anxiety disorder (e.g., the Penn State Worry Questionnaire), PTSD (e.g., the Posttraumatic Stress Disorder Diagnostic Scale), social anxiety disorder (e.g., the Social Interaction Anxiety Scale and the Social Phobia Scale), depression (e.g., the Patient Health Questionnaire and/or the Beck Depression Inventory), insomnia (e.g., the Insomnia Severity Index), as well as for screening symptoms of other complicating symptoms such as mania (e.g., the Mood Disorder Questionnaire), stress and anxiety (e.g., the Depression, Anxiety and Stress Scales and/or the Beck Anxiety Inventory), general health (e.g., the MOS SF-36 health survey questionnaire), disability (e.g., the Sheehan Disability Scale), quality of life (e.g., the Quality of Life Enjoyment and Satisfaction Questionnaire), substance abuse (e.g., the Alcohol Use Disorders Identification Test—Consumption or the Drug Abuse Screen Test), and so on.

As mentioned above, the excellent volume by Antony et al. (2001) details many disorder-specific measures of anxiety, including how to obtain copies of them. For example, the chapter describing measures for OCD includes descriptions of the Compulsive Activity Checklist, the Frost Indecisiveness Scale, the Maudsley Obsessional–Compulsive Inventory, the Obsessive–Compulsive Inventory, the Overvalued Ideas Scale, the Padua Inventory—Washington State University Revision, the Responsibility Attitude Scale, Responsibility Interpretations Questionnaire, the Thought–Action Fusion Scale, and the Yale–Brown Obsessive–Compulsive Scale. The chapter also contains brief descriptions of additional measures, such as the Brown Assessment of Beliefs Scale, the Obsessional Beliefs Questionnaire, and the Vancouver Obsessional–Compulsive Inventory, as well as brief descriptions of measures for obsessive–compulsive spectrum disorders, such as body dysmorphic disorder, trichotillomania, and tics.

Another volume in the ABCT Clinical Assessment Series, *Practitioner's Guide to Empirically-Based Measures of Depression* by Nezu, Ronan, Meadows, and McClure (2000), offers the similar advice for scales that measure the various aspects of depression. In addition, at least two other volumes in the series that are worth exploring, depending on the nature of the populations served, include *Practitioner's Guide to Empirically Based Measures of Social Skills* by Nangle, Hansen, Erdley, and Norton (2010) and *Practitioner's Guide to Empirically Based Measures of School Behavior* by Kelley, Noell, and Reitman (2003).

## GIVING FEEDBACK AND PRESENTING A CASE FORMULATION TO THE PATIENT

The final step in maximizing the potential for a positive treatment outcome involves providing feedback to the patient (as well as any other invested parties, such as the patient's significant other, key family members, and friends/coworkers). This should definitely be provided prior to the start of any treatment and most typically is provided at the session following the initial evaluation. Regardless of when it is conducted, the feedback meeting should contain several components, including (1) provision of the DSM diagnosis, with a focus on the criteria met to warrant the diagnosis of OCD, (2) brief psychoeducation about the diagnosis, including a presentation of the case formulation (see below), (3) treatment options (including medications), along with a brief description of evidence-based and pros and cons of each treatment option and the estimated course of treatment, (4) the prognosis, along with factors influencing it, and (5) time for feedback and questions.

# CASE FORMULATION

As emphasized throughout this chapter, after conducting a structured diagnostic evaluation and a thorough general clinical evaluation, it is important to develop a detailed case formulation. The case formulation is best seen as a working hypothesis that synthesizes all of the information gathered in the intake evaluation (including the empirically based self-report measures) and frames it in terms of the cognitive-behavioral model of OCD. In so doing, it provides (typically in either a brief narrative or a flowchart) a summary of the patient's symptoms, the suspected origins of the symptoms, the triggers that currently activate the symptoms, and a description of the psychopathological mechanisms that are believed to generate and maintain the patient's symptoms as well as any additional factors (e.g., interpersonal, situational, comorbid conditions) that are thought to be influencing the patient's disorder. In so doing, the case formulation becomes a "blueprint" for the goals of treatment, which will then target the psychopathological mechanisms underlying the disorder and other complicating factors, in an effort to reduce the patient's symptoms and help the patient achieve a better quality of life.

Thus, by generating the case formulation and sharing it with the patient (and other relevant parties) before the start of treatment, you have the opportunity to reflect to the patient an understanding of the patient's experience, present a hypothesis about what's maintaining the patient's symptoms, encourage a collaborative therapeutic relationship soliciting the patient's feedback, and increase motivation and hope by presenting an explanation of how the treatment will target the maintaining factors to help the patient feel better. However, the initial case formulation should be considered only a "rough draft" and, as such, should be constantly revisited and revised as the treatment progresses (or stalls) or new information is obtained.

## Sample Case Formulation

Scott is a 40-year-old, single, Jewish American male who lives alone in an apartment in New York City and works as a manager in a local department store. He was self-referred for therapy owing to a recent exacerbation in his symptoms that has caused his work performance to slide. On the initial visit, his chief complaint was: "I can't stop myself from checking things over and over again. I've tried to control it on my own but it's been getting worse and I need to try something new."

[Context in which the OCD developed/predisposing factors.] Scott reported that his mother was "a major worrier" [psychological/biological vulnerability] and his paternal grandmother and paternal aunt suffered from panic attacks and agoraphobia [biological vulnerability]. In addition, he reported that his father was a "neat freak" and "germaphobe" who was always arranging things around the house and always washing his hands and doing laundry during the patient's developmental years [psychological/biological vulnerability]. As a result, Scott noted that he came to learn that the world was a dangerous place [overestimation of threat] and, unless he took certain measures [inflated responsibility], he would be vulnerable [overestimation of likelihood] to harm. As a result, he learned to focus his efforts on monitoring for potential threats [information processing bias] and, as a precaution, unless he could be absolutely certain [intolerance of uncertainty], to assume the worst, so he would not be caught off guard [maladaptive metacognition].

[Context in which the OCD worsened.] Scott reported having these beliefs for as long as he could remember, but he emphasized that they did not really interfere with his day-to-day living until approximately 2 months ago, when he was promoted to manager at his work [precipitating factor]. As a result of the promotion, he was given additional responsibilities and tasks, which included being in charge of locking up the department store at the end of the night [trigger] and setting the security alarm [trigger]. Scott noted that these two new tasks, which he had to complete at the end of the night and as the last (and only) person in the store, were the "one–two punch" that had sent his anxiety spiraling out of control. Scott explained that as he nears the end of his shift, his anxiety begins to escalate and eventually reaches a level that makes it impossible for him to concentrate on attending to the tasks at hand, especially making sure the doors are locked and the alarm is set—the two tasks he deemed most important. As a result, he often finds himself doubting the accuracy of his memory [intolerance of uncertainty] of having locked the doors and set the alarm, which makes him even more anxious.

Scott reported that he had tried to manage his anxiety in a number of ways [perpetuating factors/rituals]. These included giving the door handles an extra shake to make sure they were locked, mentally repeating a list of doors he had checked, placing colored sticky dots on the doors he had locked, turning the alarm on and off several times until he felt convinced it was properly armed, and reentering the store to confirm that the alarm was set. He noted that he had even tried to cope by "assigning" the task to another staff member [avoidance] or making an excuse that he had to leave early and asking another staff member to "cover" for him at the end of the night [escape], but he was reprimanded by his supervisor for doing this and told he had to be the one to complete these tasks. Thus, with no one to help him and no way to avoid the tasks, Scott was finding himself getting increasingly anxious and needing to engage in more rituals to manage his anxiety.

Scott understood that his repeated checking behaviors were excessive and unreasonable [good insight], but stated that despite this awareness, he couldn't seem to stop himself from doing them: he feared that if he forgot just once, someone could break in and "make off" with all of their inventory [feared consequence], and he would be held responsible [appraisal of inflated responsibility]. As a result, he noted that it had reached the point where he now spends 1–2 hours at the end of the night checking all of the doors and setting and then resetting the alarm system before being able to leave. In addition, he said that most recently, he had been driving back to work in the middle of the night to check the locks and alarm one more time and had started calling the security company responsible for responding to the alarm, to ask them to check the system to make sure it was activated and working. He even mentioned that he had started to check to make sure the doors to his apartment were locked before he went to bed and before he left for work. He noted that all of this checking was starting to take a toll on his social life (he was having to cancel meetings with friends because he could not leave work) and occupational life (he was arriving at work drowsy from being up late night before) and causing him a great deal of distress.

Scott reported that he had not told his family about his struggles [avoidance] out of concern that they would worry about him [maladaptive cognition]. Similarly, he had not told his friends, coworkers, or boss about his struggles [avoidance], out of a fear that they would either think he was crazy and would not want to be friends with him, or, in the case of his boss, fire him [maladaptive cognitions]. Instead, Scott's sole coping strategy has been to use more and more rituals to manage his anxiety.

The rituals are undoubtedly reinforcing because they serve to reduce Scott's discomfort temporarily [negative reinforcement]. Unfortunately, engaging in these rituals also serves to strengthen the importance of the obsessive thoughts (e.g., I've not set the alarm properly, I've forgotten to lock one of the doors) and appraisals (I felt anxious because something bad was going to happen, I would have been responsible, etc.), as well as his maladaptive cognitions about anxiety (e.g., if I do not engage in rituals, my anxiety will spiral out of control). As a result of this inflated importance, Scott has started to pay more attention in key situations (e.g., locking up at the end of the night) that trigger his obsessions and, consequently, has been experiencing the intrusive thoughts with greater frequency and has been feeling more and more anxious. This in turn has led Scott to resort to more compulsions, thus forming a vicious cycle [cognitive-behavioral model]

Scott is aware that his system has not been working and is interfering with his enjoyment and satisfaction in life. He is also aware that if he does not make a change he will be at risk of losing his promotion or even his job and spending even less time with his friends and family. As a result, he is very motivated to try CBT and is willing to do what it takes to get his life back under control again. He has realistic expectations and goals for the therapy, despite never having been in treatment before.

---

### TAKE–HOME MESSAGE

Along with conducting a brief Phone Screen (see Appendix B, Form 1) and structured diagnostic evaluation (see Chapter 4), it is important to place the patient's presenting symptoms in the context of both his current living environment and life history in order to prepare him for treatment and to maximize the potential for a positive treatment outcome. Conducting a general clinical evaluation can help to do this and, when combined with the information obtained from a more structured diagnostic evaluation and other evidence-based (clinician-administered or self-report) assessment measures, can be used to create a comprehensive biopsychosocial case formulation that will prepare the patient for treatment and to maximize the potential for a positive treatment outcome. Althoughg each of these two phases was described separately, they can in fact be combined in any way the clinician deems appropriate (e.g., one longer session and/or reversed in order of administration).

# CHAPTER 6

# Comprehensive Plan for Treating Obsessive–Compulsive Disorder

## *Overview*

This section of the book sets forth a proposed plan for treating OCD using a cognitive-behavioral approach that can be delivered in 16 weekly, individual, 50- to 60-minute sessions. Given the current health care environment and typical patterns in which patients are scheduled, this format appears to be the best fit for most outpatient clinical practices. Many of the treatment protocols used in the efficacy and effectiveness research from which the expert consensus treatment guidelines for OCD were derived employed a more intense course of treatment (e.g., twice-weekly, "double" sessions of 90–120 minutes, delivered over 8–10 weeks or even daily, "double" sessions, delivered over three consecutive weeks, along with the use of several planned brief phone sessions). Treatment outcome studies, however, have also been able to demonstrate success using once-weekly, individual sessions of "standard" length (i.e., 45–50 minutes), such as the one described in the following chapters.

At its foundation, this treatment plan employs Ex/RP, which expert consensus considers to be the "gold-standard" psychological treatment for patients with OCD. As is the case with exposure-based treatments for other anxiety disorders, in Ex/RP the goal is for patients to ultimately face the feared triggers (e.g., situations, images, or objects), without engaging in any of the rituals and/or safety behaviors they have become used to employing to manage their anxiety or to "prevent" negative consequences from occurring. When conducted properly, Ex/RP is a powerful and robust psychological intervention that not only utilizes habituation but also creates the context for emotional processing and new learning to occur.

With Ex/RP at its heart, the treatment plan that follows is appropriate for all patients with OCD, regardless of how long they have been symptomatic, the severity of the disorder, or their type of OCD symptoms. However, you should be sure to *customize the treatment to fit the patient* (see Chapter 5, "Case Formulation" section), rather than try to *force the patient to fit the therapy*. In other words, you should build an idiosyncratic Ex/RP model for each patient, which, at various times, will likely need to be adjusted, along with the treatment goals, the interventions being used, and the pacing of the treatment, to address the patient's specific life situation. For example, you may need to make adjustments at various times during the treatment in order to take into account a patient's varying degree of insight, motivation, psychiatric and medical comorbidity, and psychosocial stressors. A thorough intake evaluation, detailed case formulation, sound clinical judgment, and, above all, clinical flexibility should allow you to maximize the results of this core treatment plan by tailoring it to meet the unique needs of each individual patient.

Ex/RP for OCD has traditionally included several components: (1) introducing the general model and principles of CBT, (2) introducing the CBT model of OCD, (3) providing psychoeducation on the symptoms of OCD, (4) daily monitoring the OCD symptoms, (5) creating a hierarchy for Ex/RP, (6) engaging in Ex/RP, and (7) preventing relapse. As mentioned in previous chapters, however, expert consensus guidelines suggest beginning treatment of OCD with either CBT alone or a combination of CBT and a medication. As such, you should account for the role (or lack thereof) that medications will play in the treatment when crafting the case formulation. In addition, if the patient is already taking a medication at intake, it is important that you consider their potential effects (positive and negative) on the implementation of this treatment plan.

As mentioned in previous chapters, along with Ex/RP, a number of other approaches can be of benefit to patients with OCD. For example, the cognitive model of OCD places a greater emphasis on the key role that faulty appraisals (e.g., an inflated sense of personal responsibility related to events that may cause harm to either themselves or others) play in perpetuating the symptoms. As such, cognitive approaches to OCD often include specific techniques that aim to address and correct these faulty appraisals (e.g., by helping the person identify, test, and evaluate the veracity of his appraisals) that a good cognitive-behavioral therapist would be wise to know, even if primarily focusing on implementing Ex/RP. In addition, despite the different emphases found in the behavioral and cognitive models of OCD, in practice, many clinicians ultimately choose to combine Ex/RP with cognitive techniques.

As a result, this treatment planner will include several examples of cognitive techniques, as well as some techniques derived from several additional psychological approaches (e.g., metacognitive, mindfulness, acceptance and commitment, motivational enhancement), which have also been shown to be effective in treating OCD but have yet to be evaluated with the same scientific rigor as Ex/RP. However, these approaches are designed to be *optional* components of this treatment planner. As such, they may be included, in any order, with or without adaptation, or completely omitted, depending on your case formulation of the patient's OCD and how successfully the therapy progresses.

For example, some patients may struggle to understand the CBT model of OCD and thus not understand how Ex/RP can be helpful in treating their disorder and express reluctance (i.e., resistance, low motivation) to engage in the treatment. In these cases, rather than trying to force the patient to engage in the therapy, you would be better off spending more time in the initial phase of the treatment—explaining and elaborating on the CBT model and treatment rationale and exploring the patient's concerns. This will help to enhance the patient's motivation and commitment to the treatment, both of which are critical during the implementation of exposure exercises that constitute the core of the treatment—and ultimately to final treatment outcome.

Other patients with OCD may also be experiencing comorbid depression, which can interfere with the treatment by negatively impacting their ability to attend sessions regularly and/or comply with the homework assignments. In these cases, you would be better off spending time addressing the depression first—including considering a referral to a psychiatrist for a medication evaluation and involving family members, loved ones, or friends as "coaches" in the treatment—if doing so will ultimately help the patient to engage more fully in the treatment and improve the final outcome.

For other patients, the severity of their symptoms, changes and demands in their home environment, or variations in their level of insight may at some point become too challenging for them to be successfully treated using weekly appointments in an outpatient setting. For such patients, you should consider varying the dose/intensity of the sessions (e.g., multiple days per week and/or longer sessions) or collaborate with the patient to set terms under which a referral to a more intense level of care (e.g., a day program or inpatient hospital program) will be warranted.

Conversely, some experts have suggested that it may be most useful and cost effective for patients to start at the *least* intensive level of evidence-based care possible; then, should the less intensive "dosing" of therapy fail, the treatment can be "stepped up" to the next most intense level of care. For example, some patients may benefit simply from a detailed assessment and then a guided self-help format of therapy, whereas others may need more contact with a therapist, but may not have to meet weekly and could benefit from computer-assisted therapy or even a group outpatient therapy format. As a result, you may also want to consider the conditions under which a patient may start treatment meeting less than once per week and under which conditions the dose/intensity of the sessions can be deescalated (e.g., tapered down from once weekly to biweekly or shorter sessions).

Finally, some patients may progress as expected though the Ex/RP plan described in the next chapters, only to suffer a lapse or relapse at a future date. Should setback occur, you and the patient may need to extend the treatment in order to return to the case formulation and adjust it to account for whatever seemed to have led to the lapse or relapse. This may involve either a review of prior techniques that the patient has already learned that can be adapted to the new trigger or the addition of new techniques to expand the patient's skill set. Either way, a similar trigger should not have the same impact in the future.

---

## TAKE-HOME MESSAGE

Treatment planners such as this one can be of assistance by describing the core components associated with successful treatment outcomes (in this case, Ex/RP). Yet it is wise to remember that at the heart of all successful treatments is a solid case formulation—and the use of a treatment planner such as this should not preclude the creation of one. Ideally, you will learn to use Ex/RP as the backbone for treatment of OCD, while also judiciously selecting appropriate adjunctive interventions (e.g., cognitive, metacognitive, acceptance and commitment, motivational), based on the case formulation you generate at the beginning of treatment, and as the formulation is adjusted and refined in response to the data that is generated as the treatment progresses. In other words, despite aiming to start treatment using Ex/RP, the specific treatment plan you create should be customized to each patient, based on factors such as the severity of illness, diagnostic comorbidity, age, culture, and level of insight, as well as access to provider and insurance issues. In addition, you should strive to be as *flexible* as possible when structuring the treatment: adjusting the format and pace (e.g., frequency and length of sessions) to match the patient's evolving needs.

# CHAPTER 7

# Treatment Session 1

## SESSION COMPONENTS

- Check on symptoms
  - Optional: Provide and score self-report measure(s)[1]
- Feedback on the assessment phase
  - Psychoeducation on diagnosis and prognosis and case formulation
  - Psychoeducation on evidence-based treatment options
- Presentation of the CBT principles and overview of the CBT model
- Mini-motivation enhancement and commitment to the treatment
- Goals and expectations for therapy (therapist and patient) and session planning
- Questions and answers
- Homework: Rationale and assignment
- Rapport and alliance building: Feedback, summary, and a take-home message

## MATERIALS NEEDED

- Self-report measures (optional)
- Expert consensus guidelines for treatment of OCD (see Appendix A)
- Dry-erase board, easel, or clip board for you to use
- Clip board for the patient to take notes during the session
- Optional: Treatment contract
- Handouts/forms for homework (see Appendix B)
  - Self-Monitoring Forms (see Appendix B)
  - NIH Fact Sheet on Obsessive–Compulsive Disorder (see Appendix B)
  - Self-help book recommendations (optional)[2]

---

[1]A list of empirically based self-report measures for OCD and other disorders can be found in Appendix A and a copy of the Obsessive–Compulsive Inventory—Revised can be found in Appendix C (Form 11).

[2]A list of self-help books for OCD can be found in Appendix A.

# CHECK ON SYMPTOMS

Creating a structured method for tracking progress in therapy is a core component of evidence-based practice. As a result, at the start of each treatment session, at a minimum be sure to do a brief check-in with the patient on the severity of the OCD symptoms and how the patient believes he has been managing the symptoms since the last session. For example, you can ask the patient to rate, on average since the last session, using 0–10 scales (1) how severe the OCD symptoms have been, (2) the amount of effort he has made in trying to manage the symptoms, and (3) the level of success he has had in managing the symptoms. You can then enter these scores into a spreadsheet program (e.g., Microsoft Excel), and chart or graph them each week to show to the patient.

Reviewing the ratings each week allows you and your patient to discuss how the treatment is progressing. If you note improvements, ask the patient why he thinks his symptoms have improved (e.g., due to the amount of effort he has put into the treatment and/or an increase in his ability to manage the symptoms). If there has been no improvement in the ratings or the patient reports a deterioration, then you and the patient can explore why the patient believes this to be the case, and you can either normalize this experience (if no apparent treatment-interfering factors can be elicited) or problem-solve as needed (e.g., assess and enhance motivation, review the homework assigned and rationale for consistently working hard between sessions to improve treatment outcome, problem-solve treatment-interfering factors, reconceptualize the case).

## Optional: Provide and Score Self-Report Measure(s)

In the spirit of maintaining an evidence-based practice, it can also be useful to have the patient complete a brief, empirically based, self-report measure of OCD (e.g., the OCI-R[3]; included in Appendix C, Form 11). As mentioned earlier in this treatment planner, using an empirically based self-report measure has many benefits, including the fact that it allows for (1) the objective and structured (i.e., valid and reliable) measurement of the symptoms of OCD, (2) comparisons to be made with established norms, (3) the objective evaluation of treatment outcome (if administered at least at pre- and posttreatment, and (4) the normalization of symptoms (i.e., seeing their symptoms listed on an assessment measure "tells" patients that they are not alone in experiencing the symptoms).

In addition, as many of these self-report measures can be completed in less than 5 minutes, they can be used as treatment "process" measures (e.g., given at each session, every few sessions, or at a predefined time interval) without having any significant negative impact on the session time. In other words, if used in a manner similar to the subjective check on symptoms described above (e.g., scored immediately), this will allow you and the patient to review when and where progress (or the lack thereof) is being made in the therapy, as well as to determine which aspects of the OCD are still in need of improvement/targeting before terminating the treatment—but in a more objective way.

When used properly (e.g., results are shared without judgment), it can also help you and the patient be more accountable for the treatment outcome. In so doing, when the results are positive

---

[3]The Administration and Scoring Sheet for the OCI-R in Appendix C should be used by the clinician and should *not* be provided to the patient.

(e.g., the patient can see objectively that scores are changing in the desired direction/progress is being made), it can reinforce efforts made, increase motivation, and enhance treatment compliance. When the results are negative (e.g., the scores did not change or indicate an increase in symptoms), it can encourage the shared exploration of possible negative contributing factors, enhancement of problem-solving skills, and normalization of the nonlinear path of treatment progress.

## FEEDBACK ON THE ASSESSMENT PHASE

One of the core principles of CBT involves "collaborative empiricism" (i.e., creating and maintaining an active collaboration between the patient and therapist in which both agree to act as scientists with respect to understanding and treating the patient's symptoms/disorder). In other words, you and the patient agree to act as a team, with you being the expert on the theory and thus taking the lead on the case conceptualization and the patient being the expert on her life and thus taking the lead on "testing out" the theory between sessions (i.e., engaging in homework exercises). As such, in the spirit of collaboration, if feedback was not provided as the final step at the end of the initial evaluation, then the initial step in treatment can involve providing feedback on the assessment phase to the patient (as well as any other invested parties, such as a partner or family member).

Be sure that the feedback includes a summary of the findings from the diagnostic assessment, general clinical evaluation, and clinician-administered OCD-specific assessment measures, as well as the empirically based self-report measures packet that the patient completed (ideally placing his score in the context of any available norms, as well as the overall clinical picture). The feedback meeting can also contain several additional components, including providing the patient with (1) a preliminary DSM diagnosis (with a focus on the criteria met to warrant the diagnosis of OCD); (2) brief psychoeducation about the diagnosis, including a presentation of the case formulation (see Chapter 5) as well as the estimated course of treatment and prognosis; (3) a summary of evidence-based treatment options (including medications), along with a brief review of the pros and cons of each treatment option; and (4) time for the patient to ask any questions about, or provide reactions to, your findings. It is important to resolve any issues (e.g., patient disagrees with diagnosis, confusion about the treatment approach, work involved between sessions) before commencing with the treatment.

### Psychoeducation on Diagnosis and Prognosis and Case Formulation: Feedback Example

"Joan, based on the intake evaluation that I performed, I've given you the diagnosis of obsessive–compulsive disorder, or "OCD" for short. I'd like to take a moment and show you how I've come up with this diagnosis, using a book [takes out the DSM and flips to the section that contains OCD] that mental health professionals refer to when making diagnoses. Let's take a look at what it says for OCD.

"As you can see from this summary box [points to the diagnostic box in the DSM for

OCD], the unwanted and intrusive thoughts about accidentally killing someone that you've been repeatedly experiencing for the past few years are called *obsessions*, and all of the things that you have been doing each day to make sure that the people around you are safe, such as driving around the block to make sure you did not hit a pedestrian and cutting your family members' meals into tiny bite-sized portions for them, are called *compulsions*. As you may have guessed by the name, obsessions and compulsions make up the core of OCD. Can you see how they are connected? [Looks for the patient's understanding of the notion that obsessions raise anxiety and compulsions relieve it.]

"It's important for you to know that many of the symptoms you've told me about are commonly reported by most people—even those who don't have a diagnosis of OCD. [This normalizes the symptoms.] In fact, there was a study done back in 1978 that found that intrusive thoughts such as the ones you've been experiencing are almost *universal*. It's just that, for you, they have been particularly bothersome and severe—coming back again and again, making you feel very anxious, taking up so much of your time, stopping you from getting things done at home and at work, and causing tension in your relationships with your family, friends, and colleagues. That's a real shame, and in a moment, I'd like to tell you about some things we can try to help you feel better—not just in the short term, but in a way that lasts.

"Before I do that, however, I would like to point out a couple more things I found during the intake evaluation. First, while doing the structured diagnostic interview and general clinical evaluation helped me to establish your diagnosis and some of your history with OCD, I can see from the more focused interview [presents the Y-BOCS and reviews the symptom checklist] that we did last week, that you have other symptoms that would fit the diagnosis of OCD—such as when you worry that something bad will happen unless things around your house and office are properly arranged, when you get stuck needing to remember insignificant things such as phone numbers on infomercials and what you had for dinner last week, and the fact that you are so bothered by odd numbers that you need to neutralize them with even numbers. I can also see from the more focused interview that we did that you find it very difficult to resist and control the symptoms and, in fact, your score of 26 from that interview falls in the severe range of OCD.

"In addition, based on your responses to the self-report measures that I gave you, I think we should continue to monitor your mood, as you endorsed several symptoms that are commonly associated with depression [refers to the Beck Depression Inventory self-report score] as well as a number of symptoms associated with panic attacks [refers to the Panic Disorder Severity Scale self-report score]. Based on the diagnostic interview I performed, I do not think these symptoms are severe enough to warrant any additional diagnoses [e.g., major depressive disorder or panic disorder]. In fact, I have a feeling that you are experiencing these symptoms *because of your OCD* and, as a result, I think they should resolve if we can successfully treat it. However, your scores were high enough on the self-report measures to lead me to think that we should monitor these symptoms so we can keep an eye on them as we get into the treatment and make sure that they (1) do not interfere with the work we want to do on your OCD and (2) start to resolve as predicted as your OCD symptoms improve. Do you have any questions about this?

"The good news is that you don't report having any other significant issues that sometimes can complicate the treatment [instillation of hope]. For example, you noted that your health is reasonably good and that you don't have any recent medical issues. You also do not have many complicating factors in your home and work environment and in fact, to the contrary, you report that, despite there being some strain in the your relationships with your family, friends, and colleagues, you generally have a very supportive family and social network, and despite your OCD symptoms, you have managed to maintain a fairly good life for yourself [highlights strengths, resiliencies, and mitigating factors]. You also noted that it's all getting too exhausting and overwhelming and know that what you're doing is excessive and unreasonable [highlights good insight]. Given all of these factors, I think the prognosis is very good for your treatment. But before we talk about your treatment options, let's see what you think of how I've put together all of the pieces of the intake evaluation and how I think your OCD symptoms are being maintained [presents case formulation].

"[Presents predisposing factors or factors that had put the patient at risk for developing OCD.] First, you reported that both of your parents have a history of anxiety issues. In fact, you even think that they may have symptoms similar to your own (e.g., you said your mother calls every day to make sure you made it to work and if she does not hear from you, starts calling your husband to make sure you are OK, and your father has endless lists that he scribbles all over the place and always seems to be counting things). While they may or may not have OCD, can you see how they may have contributed to your having it? [Looks for the patient's awareness of her biological and psychological vulnerabilities.]

"[Presents precipitating factors or factors that appear to have triggered the onset of the OCD.] Second, you reported that you had symptoms of OCD since you were a young child that had changed over the years [e.g., used to need to tap and touch things, repeat certain phrases over and over again, and had to turn your bedroom light on and off until it felt right before you could go to sleep] but had never reached the point where they caused you significant distress, disrupted what you needed to get done, impacted your relationships, or took up a lot of time. This all seems to have changed, however, after the birth of your second child five years ago, and worsened two years ago after you discovered you had accidentally left the oven on one night. As a result, you seem to have become very concerned about the idea that you might inadvertently do something that could cause harm to someone in your family.

"[Presents perpetuating factors/rituals or factors that appear to be maintaining the OCD.] Third, you reported that, over the years, you have tried "everything under the sun" to get rid of these thoughts and the anxiety that they cause you [e.g., cutting your family members' meals into tiny bite-sized portions, arranging things around your house and office, neutralizing unlucky numbers with lucky numbers, avoiding using the oven]. While you noted that these sorts of actions have worked to give you some temporary relief [highlights the power of negative reinforcement (e.g., removal of anxiety in the short term) in perpetuating and exacerbating the rituals in the long term], have you noticed that, despite all of these attempts to make the OCD go away, it seems to have continued to bother you, and in fact has only gotten worse over the years?

"For example, now you not only are concerned that you might inadvertently do something that could cause harm to someone in your family, but also that you might inadvertently do something that could cause harm to a stranger. And you reported that you are now needing to check more and more that you have in fact not harmed anyone, which has started to interfere with your ability to get to sleep at a decent hour, get to work on time, and perhaps most ironically, is causing a heavy strain to be put on the relationships with the people you love the most and are most concerned about harming in some way. Why do you think this is the case? [Looks for the patient's insight into the perpetuating role that avoidance, rituals, and/or maladaptive appraisals play in maintaining the OCD.]

"The rituals and avoidant behaviors you have come to rely on are like a double-edged sword: while they have managed to give you some temporary relief from your fears and anxiety, they have also never let you test your fears to see if they are valid. As a result, you have come to believe that the reason nothing bad has happened is due to the fact that you have performed these rituals, thereby making it very important that you watch out for potential threats [triggers/thoughts] and then do something to neutralize these threats [rituals]. Once you decided that it was your job to look out for potential threats, you did so with more and more intensity [i.e., hypervigilance] and, in so doing, seem to have broadened your definition of what counts as a threat. You also seem to have taken the stance of betting on the worst case when you can't be certain if something is a threat [i.e., intolerance of uncertainty]—just in case [e.g., "It's better to be safe than sorry!"]. Taking all of these steps has increased the frequency in which you have noticed triggers and experienced intrusive thoughts, which in turn you have interpreted as confirmation that they must be important and that you indeed are responsible for the safety of the people around you. Ironically, this has only served to make you feel more and more anxious over time, which has led you to engage in more and more rituals to cope, etc. Does this make sense to you? [Looks for the patient's insight into the CBT model of OCD.]

"[Presents treatment rationale.] So, if everything you have felt compelled to do to fight the unwanted thoughts about you being responsible for something bad from happening to someone and get away from your anxiety has worked in the short term but inadvertently made the thoughts more powerful and anxiety stronger in the long term, what do you think you need to do to start to reverse this cycle? [Looks for the patient's insight into the rationale for Ex/RP and/or cognitive/metacognitive/acceptance-based/mindfulness interventions.]

"The good news is that we now have some very good treatment options for OCD, which have been shown in studies throughout the world to significantly reduce the symptoms of OCD in people reporting symptoms that are similar to yours [instillation of hope]. And quite often, we've seen that after the symptoms of OCD are reduced, many of the other problems that people report, such as panic attacks and depressive symptoms in your case, also improve. So, I'd like to take a moment and go over a summary of what the experts agree are the best treatments available for OCD, based on research evidence gathered from around the world. That way we can decide together on what the best course of action will be for you going forward. But before I start, do you have any questions or concerns about what I've said so far?"

## Psychoeducation on Evidence-Based Treatment Options

You can then review some of the expert consensus guidelines for OCD. This can be done using a summary from a credible source, such as the National Institute of Mental Health, the National Institute for Health and Clinical Excellence, the Agency for Healthcare Research and Quality, the website on Research-Supported Psychological Treatments by the Society of Clinical Psychology (American Psychological Association, Division 12), Evidence-Based Treatment for Children and Adolescents (American Psychological Association, Division 53), the American Psychiatric Association, PsychGuides, or A Guide to Treatments That Work. See Appendix A for specific information on how to find these resources on the Internet.

In essence, there are two main treatment options to review: (1) CBT using Ex/RP and (2) medications. When presenting these options, it is important to be balanced and objective, and stick to what the empirical literature (or expert guidelines) states. As mentioned earlier, one way to do this is to present the pros and cons of each intervention. For example, the advantages of CBT using Ex/RP over medications include (1) an equal or greater decrease in OCD symptoms in a treatment package that is (2) relatively brief in duration (be sure to give an estimate of the number of sessions—in this case, 16), and (3) has a much greater durability (i.e., much lower relapse rate than medications), (4) without any side effects (unless one counts the short-term increase in anxiety as patients engage in the Ex/RP portion of the treatment). The advantages of medications over CBT include the following: (1) they do not require patients to face their fears (i.e., engage in exposure) as part of the treatment, (2) they involve less effort than CBT to implement (not required to learn a new set of skills, no homework between visits, etc.), (3) they are easier to access than CBT (it is difficult to find a therapist trained in Ex/RP), and (4) they are potentially less costly (at least in the short term). Medications also have some disadvantages: (1) they often produce unpleasant side effects and (2) they must be taken continually to maintain treatment gains, which leads them (3) to be more costly than CBT in the long term or (4) to show a much higher relapse rate than CBT if they are discontinued.

## PRESENTATION OF THE CBT PRINCIPLES AND OVERVIEW OF THE CBT MODEL

Once the patient has been provided with the evidence-based treatment options, it is often a good idea to provide her with a brief introduction to CBT (focusing on the core principles that separate it from other psychotherapy approaches), as well as an overview of the general CBT model. Some key principles of CBT include that it (1) separates etiological factors from perpetuating factors (i.e., asserts that what causes and what maintains a problem can be two very different things), (2) places an emphasis on the here-and-now, (3) attempts to be brief and time-limited in scope, (4) uses an agenda so that each session is structured and goal-oriented, (5) is skills-based, (6) includes homework exercises, (7) assumes that symptoms can and will return and therefore builds relapse prevention strategies into the treatment, (8) has as its goal to help patients become their own therapist by the end of the treatment and, perhaps most importantly, as mentioned earlier, (9) takes a "collaborative empiricism" stance in which an active collaboration between the patient and therapist is sought, with both being willing to take a scientific approach to understanding and addressing the patient's symptoms.

After presenting the principles of CBT, it can also be useful to provide the patient with an overview of the general CBT model. The goal here is to emphasize that CBT is based on a theoretical model that breaks all situations down into the three major modalities that contribute to our daily experiences: feelings, actions, and thoughts. The CBT model also proposes that each of these three modalities is equally important and that each modality is inextricably interconnected with the other two. As such, CBT utilizes the bidirectional relationship that exists between feelings, actions, and thoughts in order to help patients decrease negative affective states (e.g., anxious, depressed) and attain a better quality of life. In so doing, the CBT model does not ignore feelings, but rather acknowledges the challenge of creating emotional change directly, and instead targets thoughts and actions in order to alter emotions indirectly.

For many patients, these concepts can best be illustrated by using a drawing of the CBT triangle (see Figure 7.1). This can be done on a dry-erase board, flip chart, or writing pad. Regardless of the method used to illustrate the CBT triangle, it is helpful to (1) walk the patient through this model using a style that is interactive rather than didactic, (2) explain the basic theory first and then illustrate it using a specific example from the patient's life, and (3) have patients copy it down on a notepad for themselves as you present it. Be sure to answer any questions the patient may have about it before moving on.

## MINI–MOTIVATION ENHANCEMENT AND COMMITMENT TO THE TREATMENT

While many patients seek treatment for themselves and enter into treatment with a high level of motivation, others may have either been pushed into treatment by concerned family members, friends, or colleagues and/or may be ambivalent about engaging in Ex/RP. Ideally, the topics of motivation and readiness to change will have been initiated during the initial phone contact (see Chapter 4). Often, however, motivation and readiness wax and wane, and as a result, need to be revisited before, during, and after treatment.

Even if the patient appears to be motivated enough to begin treatment immediately, it is often a good idea to conduct a mini-motivational enhancement and obtain the patient's commitment to the treatment; interventions to increase motivation can improve treatment retention and engagement and therefore ultimately, outcome. A mini-motivational enhancement involves taking a nondirective, nonjudgmental, and nonconfrontational stance while engaging the patient

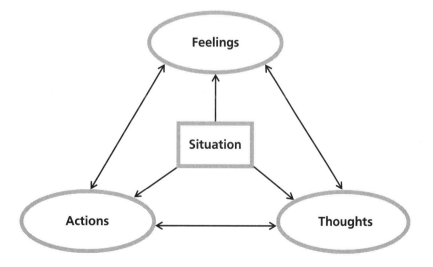

**FIGURE 7.1.** The general CBT model.

in a discussion of the costs and benefits of not beginning treatment and therefore continuing to manage the OCD in the same way (i.e., maintaining the status quo), versus the costs and benefits of beginning treatment and learning to manage the OCD in a new way (i.e., making a change). In addition to the psychological consequences, the patient can also be encouraged to consider the social, occupational, familial, and medical consequences of each decision. It is often helpful to use a tool such as a Decisional Balance Worksheet (see Figure 7.2 for a sample and Appendix B, Form 2, for a blank worksheet) to capture the main arguments for and against each decision, as patients may need to return to this worksheet throughout the treatment, whenever their motivation begins to wane. Patients may also be asked how having OCD fits with their values and goals in life, including the impact that the time they spend occupied by obsessive thoughts, engaging in rituals, and avoiding the triggers has on their mood, esteem, energy, and social and occupational functioning.

After working through a decisional balance to enhance the patient's motivation to change, it is useful to get some form of commitment from the patient. Committing means acting in the direction of what is important to you even in the presence of obstacles. Thus, commitment can be enhanced through a clarification of why it would be important to the patient, along with the

| | Benefits/Pros (short term and long term) | Costs/Cons (short term and long term) |
|---|---|---|
| **Do not make a change** (e.g., "Do not give Ex/RP a try and continue to manage my OCD the same way I always have.") | • Don't have to face my fears<br>• Save money<br>• Less work/effort required | • Continue doing my rituals<br>• Continue feeling anxious<br>• Family remains annoyed<br>• Less time for work— already on probation— could get fired<br>• Less time with my friends |
| **Make a change** (e.g., "Give Ex/RP a try so I can learn to manage my OCD in new way.") | • Freedom from my fears<br>• Won't feel controlled by my thoughts and triggers<br>• Won't have to avoid things<br>• Will no longer feel ashamed<br>• Won't need to lie about or hide my symptoms<br>• Will have more time to do the things I want to do in life<br>• Will have better relationships | • Will have to work hard<br>• Will feel anxious<br>• Worst fears might come true<br>• Expensive |

**FIGURE 7.2.** Sample Decisional Balance Worksheet.

setting of specific goals, and an open and honest discussion of the challenges that lie ahead. In addition, you can explain the importance of being willing to consider new ways to approach the symptoms—many of which may initially feel uncomfortable or wrong and thus make the patient more anxious in the short term—as he goes against his instincts and learns to question beliefs he may have held for years. At times, it may even be useful to draft a treatment "contract" that includes an overview of the treatment and the therapist's and patient's goals and expectations for therapy (which are covered in the next section). If a treatment contact is used, it should have specific, observable expectations, along with explicit connections of these goals to valued areas in the patient's life (e.g., "If I reduce my rituals, even by an hour each day to start, I can spend that time with my children"). If necessary, it should also have specific consequences for violations of expectations. Both parties should sign it, along with a witness (if available), and the patient should be given a copy.

## GOALS AND EXPECTATIONS FOR THERAPY (THERAPIST AND PATIENT) AND SESSION PLANNING

Once the patient is motivated and committed to starting the treatment, it is important to present *your* expectations of the patient, as well as to elicit, clarify and, if necessary, correct the patient's expectations of *you* (and the treatment plan). Standard expectations for you to emphasize would be the importance of the patient (1) following the principle of collaborative empiricism (i.e., being scientists together), (2) maintaining an open and honest communication style, (3) working hard during each session and between sessions, and (4) getting family members or other close friends involved. Discuss with patients any rules about attendance, including how lateness and missed appointments will be handled, and remind patients that, in order to maximize the power of the treatment, they will be expected to begin striving to prevent rituals, decrease safety behaviors, and eliminate avoidances fairly early on—all while also setting goals that serve to move them toward the things they value most in life.

It is also useful to remind the patient of the relatively short-term nature of this treatment (e.g., 16 weekly, individual, 50- to 60-minute sessions) and, whenever possible, plan out (i.e., schedule) the entire course of treatment (or as many sessions as possible) in advance. This emphasizes to the patient the principles of CBT being both a brief and time-limited treatment, and will help keep your sessions focused on the treatment goals each week. It also allows you and the patient to become aware of any potential scheduling challenges to the treatment and to make a plan for how these challenges will be addressed, right from the start. As many patients now carry smart phones or similar devices, scheduling ahead should be relatively simple. In the event that the patient does not have a smart phone, tablet, or laptop computer with a calendar function, calendar-style pages can be printed from most word processors or downloaded for free from many sites on the Internet,[4] and the sessions can then be planned out on paper. In addition, if you plan on conducting any phone sessions between the office visits, they may also be scheduled at this time.

---

[4]Entering the words "free calendar template" into Google returns more than 82 million results.

# QUESTIONS AND ANSWERS

Finally, as this session presented a great deal of information to the patient (e.g., feedback on the assessment, case formulation, rationale for treatment, treatment options, presentation of the CBT principles, overview of the CBT model, decisional balance, goals and expectations for therapy), it is useful to allow time for questions before assigning homework and wrapping up the session. In addition, it is often useful to preemptively address some of the more frequently raised concerns by patients. These concerns are listed and discussed below, as well as on a patient handout in Appendix B, Common Questions and Answers about OCD, Form 3.

## Common Questions and Answers about OCD

For many patients, entering into treatment is a big step and comes with a lot of questions. This discussion (and in handout form in Appendix B, Form 3) is designed to provide your patients with answers to the most common questions they may have about their OCD.

### *Question:* Can I expect to fully eliminate all of my OCD symptoms?

*Answer:* No! It is *normal* for most people to experience some *symptoms* of OCD. Yet, experiencing some symptoms of OCD does not mean you have a disorder! Symptoms only become a disorder when they cause a lot of (1) distress, (2) disruption, or (3) disability in your work, home, or social life. As a result, the goal of treatment is to help you learn how to *manage* your OCD symptoms more effectively. The research suggests that on average, you can expect a 60–70% improvement in your symptom severity if you fully participate in and complete the treatment.

### *Question:* Is homework really necessary?

*Answer:* Yes! CBT is unlike other types of talk therapy for this very reason. In CBT the assigning of homework is seen as essential in order for you to (1) practice building the skills you are taught in each session, (2) gather evidence to test out predictions you make in each session, (3) demonstrate that the same rules apply to life inside and outside of your therapist's office, and (4) help you learn to do the treatment on your own—without the aid of your therapist. The research is clear here: if you do not complete your homework assignments, you will not do as well in this treatment.

### *Question:* The CBT model seems too simple! Isn't OCD more complicated than that?

*Answer:* Perhaps the model seems simple, and yes, there are many competing theories about what causes and maintains OCD. But the model does not have to be complex to be effective. And simple does not mean easy. Psychological change requires two big things: insight and awareness into the problem and a willingness and commitment to do what it takes to change it. While CBT takes a simple approach, breaking down what you need to focus on into two main categories (find a new way to deal with your thoughts and change what you've been doing in response to your triggers), it still takes a while to learn how to spot your triggers, understand how your reactions and interpretations of the triggers generate your anxiety, and realize when you're engaging in rituals. It takes a great deal of courage and conviction to break the cycle.

### Question: Is *full* ritual prevention really necessary? Can't I just keep a couple of rituals?

*Answer*: Yes, full ritual prevention is really necessary. To engage in partial ritual prevention is a bit like working really hard to throw buckets of water on a fire, only to throw on the occasional jug of gasoline: in the end, the fire will keep on burning! Or think of it like removing the weeds in a garden. If you leave one or two weeds, it's only a matter of time before they start to take over again. In other words, at best, engaging in occasional rituals can dampen the impact of the treatment and prolong it unnecessarily, and at worst, engaging in occasional rituals can interfere with the new learning that is necessary to change the way you see your symptoms and set you up for a potential relapse after treatment is terminated. If you really want to maintain some of your rituals, it may mean that you have not fully understood the CBT model or treatment explanation, or that you have some special rules for certain triggers or thoughts, or are still not quite sure whether this treatment is right for you. If this is the case, you should speak with your therapist about it before starting the treatment.

### Question: Surely some of my fears are based in reality?

*Answer*: Of course! The themes of the fearsome thoughts that people with OCD experience have been found to be the *exact same* as those experienced by people who do not have OCD. The only difference is that people with OCD experience these fearsome thoughts much more frequently, intensely, and for longer periods of time. This happens because people with OCD often interpret these thoughts in ways that people without OCD do not. For example, people with OCD cannot seem to tolerate the uncertainty about which fears are based in reality and which are not as well as people without OCD. The treatment aims at correcting this intolerance of uncertainty through Ex/RP. By exposing yourself to your fears while preventing yourself from engaging in the rituals that are often performed to create more certainty (e.g., checking to make sure the stove is turned off), you will gradually learn to tolerate uncertainty more and more and you will not need to ritualize in order to feel better. This is why facing your fears and learning to tolerate your anxious feelings are *necessary* components of this treatment.

### Question: Are you sure nothing bad will happen (to me or my loved ones) if I do this treatment?

*Answer*: Yes and no. Although this treatment has been studied for many years in patients around the world diagnosed with OCD and has been recommended as the treatment of choice for OCD by experts in the fields of psychiatry and psychology, you can never *guarantee* that bad things won't happen in life. In fact, it is quite the opposite: eventually bad things happen in *all* of our lives—and so instead of spending so much of your time and effort trying to avoid thoughts about them or prevent them from happening, you must learn a *new way* to deal with your thoughts about them. This treatment will help you to *test out* whether your rituals are really preventing bad things from happening and to feel more confident in your ability to determine when something is actually posing a serious threat to you or a loved one.

### Question: How certain are you that I will see a positive result?

*Answer:* It depends on what you mean by a positive result. As mentioned above, the research suggests that on average, you can expect a 60–70% improvement in your symptom severity if you fully complete the treatment. But it's really more than just completing the treatment: one of the biggest factors in maximizing the results is the amount of work you do—in each session as well as between sessions to develop the skills necessary to become your own CBT therapist.

### Question: Have you ever treated anyone like me before? From what I've read, my symptoms don't seem common. Are you sure they will they respond to this approach?

*Answer:* Just as no two people are the same, no two patients are exactly the same. There are more common symptoms and less common symptoms of OCD. However, even if the symptoms are not common and do not fit neatly into any of the classic themes, the power of the CBT model of OCD is in the fact that it can be used to explain how *any* symptom of OCD is maintained—which can then lead to the successful treatment of that symptom.

## Homework: Rationale and Assignment

At this point, as the session is winding down, it becomes important to introduce the concept of homework and discuss in detail the rationale, purpose, and importance of completing it. It is then advisable to collaborate with the patient on determining the homework assignment for the upcoming week and designing a method for recording the results so that the assignment can be reviewed in the next session. This also allows the patient to have a record of the work she completed during the treatment, which can then be reviewed after treatment terminates.

First, remind the patient that CBT is a skills-based treatment and, as such, requires practice both within and between the sessions. Therefore, the purpose of homework is to provide the patient with an opportunity to build a skill and/or learn something new about her disorder. It is not meant to be like a school assignment (completed for you), but rather, it is meant to be completed for the benefit of the patient (with you only reviewing it to make sure concepts are being understood and learned and to give guidance, if necessary).

Inform the patient that research has shown that completion of homework between sessions is an *essential component* in enhancing treatment outcome. The facts are clear: patients who do work between sessions have better outcomes and achieve them faster than patients who do not do the homework. Warn the patient that at times she may struggle to complete the homework assignments, which is normal, especially at the start of treatment. Inform the patient that the learning comes from the struggle, and therefore the most important thing is to continually strive to give 100% effort to complete it.

Difficulty in completing homework assignments may be due to a variety of factors, such as an unclear understanding of the rationale, uncertainty about the usefulness of the assignment, confusion over the task assigned, and a lack of familiarity about how to complete it. Therefore, you can take several steps to increase the likelihood of the patient's success (i.e., "compliance") with the homework assignments. First and foremost, be sure to allocate enough time in the session to present a rationale for assigning homework—both in general (i.e., this rationale section) at the start of treatment and then again before each specific instance of assigning it. In addition, it should be collaboratively designed, with input from the patient not only being allowed, but requested, on everything from the general homework task to the specifics of how the task will be carried out and recorded. In this way, the patient will see it as useful and important and will be invested in completing it. Once designed, provide the patient with a written description of the current home-work assignment, along with instructions and an in-session demonstration on how to complete it. Finally, allow time for questions and answers about it.[5]

For this (first) treatment session, at a minimum, the homework should involve having the patient begin to increase his awareness of his OCD symptoms, so that the treatment can be tailored to the symptoms he is experiencing difficulty with in the here-and-now. Most often, a self-monitoring assignment can serve this function. A sample completed Self-Monitoring Form is included in Figure 7.3, and a blank copy of the Self-Monitoring Form, Form 4, can be found in Appendix B.

In addition to self-monitoring, the homework from this first session might include (1) having the patient review the notes taken during the session and/or return with a summary of the main points and any questions that arose while he was reviewing them; (2) providing the patient with a psychoeducational handout on OCD (e.g., the NIH Fact Sheet on Obsessive–Compulsive Behavior[6]) to review and return with a written summary of the main points and/or written list of any questions that arose while reading it; and (3) providing the patient with a self-help book sug-gestion (e.g., *Stop Obsessing!: How to Overcome Your Obsessions and Compulsions* by Edna Foa and Reid Wilson [2001] and/or *Overcoming Obsessive Thoughts: How to Gain Control of Your OCD* by Christine Purdon and David Clark [2005]; see Appendix A) and asking the patient to purchase it before the next session and ideally, read the first chapter and write a summary of the main points and/or a list of any questions that arose while reading it.

If you plan on assigning a self-help book, it should be noted that increasingly patients are downloading electronic versions of books to their smart phones or e-book readers (e.g., Kindle, Nook, iPad). As such, it would be good to have the patient do this in session, so that you can make sure he orders the correct book. If the book is not available in digital form or if your patient does not have an e-reader, it can be helpful to have a few extra copies of your favorite self-helps books available in your office, which you can then loan to your patient in order to expedite the process of obtaining the book. Of course, before assigning any self-help book for homework, be sure to read it yourself, to make sure you agree with the message it sends and you can answer any questions that the patient has about it. A list of self-help books for OCD can be found in Appendix A.

---

[5] The rising popularity of smart phones and the lowering costs of data plans have led to the creation and proliferation of applications ("apps") that will likely play an increasing role in treatment of psychological disorders. Many apps are being created with CBT themes, and several of these CBT apps are now directly targeting OCD. Although many of these apps have yet to be empirically examined, at a minimum, they should make certain homework assignments (e.g., self-monitoring) easier to complete.

[6]See Appendix B, Form 5. Also available at *http://report.nih.gov/NIHfactsheets/Pdfs/ObsessiveCompulsiveDisorder (NIMH).pdf*.

| Trigger for the obsession (or situation you were in when you experienced the obsession) | Obsession | Interpretation (what having the obsession means to you or says about you) | Level of Anxiety or Discomfort it caused you (0–10) | Ritual/ Compulsion (what you did to feel better) | Time spent on the ritual (in minutes) or number of times you performed the ritual |
|---|---|---|---|---|---|
| Handshake with therapist | Her hands are probably dirty! | I am going to get sick and miss work! | 8 | Washed hands right after leaving her office | 10 minutes |
| Sitting on subway seat | This seat is covered in germs! | My clothes are now contaminated. I am going to make my family sick. | 9 | Removed clothes and washed them as soon as I got home. | 5 minutes |
| Buying can of soda from cafeteria | Who knows how many people have touched this can? | I am going to get sick and miss work! | 8 | Selected can from back of fridge. Wiped top thoroughly before drinking. Used a straw, just in case. | 5 minutes |

**FIGURE 7.3.** Sample Self-Monitoring Form.

## Rationale for Homework and the Self-Monitoring of Rituals: Homework Assignment Example

"I want to leave a little time for us to discuss the topic of homework. As you may have heard, in order for you to get the best results that you can out of this treatment, it is going to take a lot of work, in the times that we meet as well as in-between our visits. As a result, we need to spend some time each session focusing on creating useful 'homework' assignments for you to complete. Can you tell me why you think completing homework may lead to a better outcome? [If the patient cannot give a response that fits with the CBT principle of skills acquisition, you can remind her of this principle. Sometimes, it may be useful to use an analogy, such as comparing the learning of OCD skills to that of learning a new language or musical instrument: it takes more than a once-weekly, hour-long office visit to become fluent or proficient and the more you practice the quicker you'll see results.]

"So, we need to keep a few things in mind. First, you are not completing your homework for me! This is not like school where you need to turn in your assignments for grading. Instead, you are completing the homework for you! I am just here to review how it's going and to help you where you get stuck. The main reasons we assign homework in CBT are to gather more information on something we don't quite understand, to test out an idea that we have generated in session, or to practice a skill we have introduced in our work together. The best way to do this is to either monitor whatever it is we're trying to find out more about, design an 'experiment' that can be conducted out in the 'real world' to test out an idea we generated in session and then record the 'data' generated from the experiment and bring it back in here so we can review the results together or to have you to practice any skills that are introduced in a session. In this way, we act like a team of scientists, sharing the same goal: finding different ways to relieve you of the distress caused by your OCD.

"Often, we will come up with a theory about some aspect of your OCD in my office and then send you out to gather information or test it out in the real world. As long as you are willing to gather information or complete a test of the theory, we'll be on our way. If the test goes the way we'd expect, we will know to do more of the things that are working to your benefit; if it does not work the way we'd predict, we can adjust the theory and devise a new experiment based on the information you gather. That way, we are always refining our treatment based on what you're experiencing out in the 'real world.' But without your active participation, this simply cannot get done as quickly or as efficiently. Does this make sense?

"It is also perfectly natural for patients to struggle with doing the homework—especially at the beginning of treatment. After all, if it were that easy, you would not likely need to come to treatment in the first place. There are, however, some things we can do to increase your likelihood of success. Can you think of anything that would help ensure the homework is a success? [You can note the following points: (1) saving enough time each session to review what was done and create a new assignment, (2) collaborating on the assignment, (3) having written instructions on how to complete the specific assignment(s) each week, (4) doing an in-session demonstration of it—including how to record it, (5) agreeing that it is useful, (6) connecting it to the broader treatment goal(s), (7) planning when and where it will be done, (8) anticipating any potential roadblocks in getting it done and problem-solving how to overcome them, (9) being consistent, and (10) starting small.]"

The patient may also want to enlist the help of a family member or friend as a coach in order to complete the homework. This is often useful but should only be used as an augmentation strategy, for the goal is to have the patient increase his sense of self-efficacy (versus dependence). Therefore, the coach should be educated about how best to help (encourage and remind vs. coerce or give reassurance) in order to maximize the benefits and minimize the costs of using one. If you will also be acting as a coach between sessions (i.e., offering phone support sessions), the rules (e.g., frequency, length, and format) of these should also be agreed upon at this time.

"For this week, rather than try to change what you've been doing when it comes to your OCD, I thought it would be important for us to get a good, detailed, look at your current OCD symptoms and patterns. This way, we can see just how much of your day is being taken up by your obsessions and compulsions at the moment, and use these data for monitoring your progress during the treatment. It also will make you more aware of your triggers, which can help us fine-tune your treatment. How does this sound?

"So, can we agree that your first task should be to monitor your OCD symptoms, each and every day, with the goal of increasing your awareness of your specific triggers and OCD symptoms this week? This is not always an easy task, even though it sounds quite simple. Let's go over some tips on how to monitor them. I have a sample form [hands a copy of the Self-Monitoring Form (see Appendix B, Form 4) to the patient] that you can use, if it will make things easier. Or, if you want, we can create a new form that we feel will best suit your needs. Either way, this task will call on you to record the symptoms in writing—using either a sheet of paper or a computer or smart phone application [e.g., the 'Notes' app in the iPhone]. Let's do an entry together, just to make sure we're on the same page about how to complete it."

If the patient agrees that this is a useful assignment and can connect it to the broader goal of reducing the OCD severity, you should give a copy of the Self-Monitoring Form to the patient (see Appendix B, Form 4), along with tips for making the monitoring easier (e.g., keep the form around her at all times, complete immediately after engaging in a ritual, keep entries brief). Review the form with the patient and make sure to address any questions she has about the assignment and do an in-session demonstration of how she should complete it. Anticipate any potential roadblocks in getting it done before the next session and problem-solve how to overcome them.

If the patient does not agree that this would be a useful assignment and/or cannot connect it to the broader treatment goal(s), you should address these issues before moving ahead. Sometimes a review of the rationale or model will help. At other times, a modification of the task may increase the patient's willingness to try it. As long as it is increasing the patient's awareness of his OCD symptoms, it should be considered. In any event, the patient's resistance should be discussed and addressed before moving ahead—as simply insisting that the patient complete the assignment will not likely be effective and would violate the collaborative nature of the treatment.

## RAPPORT AND ALLIANCE BUILDING: FEEDBACK, SUMMARY, AND TAKE-HOME MESSAGE

Despite being protocol-driven, the treatment of OCD still relies on a solid case conceptualization, good rapport, and a strong working alliance between patient and therapist to maximize the results. Therefore, building rapport and forging a strong working alliance with the patient are critical to treatment success. Ideally, rapport will have been building from the initial phone contact, throughout the assessment, by providing feedback and sharing the case conceptualization during this first treatment session—including ending with the collaborative generation of the homework assignment mentioned in the previous paragraph.

An additional way to enhance rapport is by eliciting feedback from the patient and giving it to the patient (if necessary), summarizing (in turns) what the session was about and, based on this agreed-on summary, clarifying and agreeing on the message (i.e., principle/theme/lesson) the patient plans to "take home" with her (i.e., based on what was covered this week, what will she now do differently in the world?). In this session, it can be helpful to elicit feedback from the patient on what you have presented in terms of the diagnosis and formulation, prognosis, treatment options, rationale for a CBT approach and the CBT model, expectations for therapy, and first homework assignment.

## TAKE-HOME MESSAGE FROM TREATMENT SESSION 1

Treatment Session 1 serves as a "bridge" between the assessment and treatment phases. As such, you may be tempted to consider it less important than the other sessions (e.g., the initial evaluation, the start of exposure). In many ways, however, this may be the *most important* of all the sessions, for it allows you to present/confirm a clear diagnostic picture to the patient and provide critical information on the diagnosis, prognosis, and evidence-based treatments for OCD. Recall that, on average, it takes 14 to 17 years from the time OCD begins for people to get the right treatment. As a result, by providing this information to patients, you will be starting them on a path that they have long been searching for, and have the opportunity to instill hope and confidence in you and the treatment by presenting a detailed, specific rationale behind CBT. You can also go a long way toward enhancing the patient's motivation and commitment to the treatment by providing a clear overview of the CBT model, addressing any ambivalence (using a decisional balance, if necessary), and agreeing on the expectations for therapy. Finally, the structure and tone of future sessions can be set by planning ahead, discussing the importance of homework, and building rapport and alliance through soliciting feedback, agreeing on a summary of the session, and providing a take-home message.

# CHAPTER 8

# Treatment Session 2

## SESSION COMPONENTS

- Check on symptoms
  - Optional: Provide and score self-report measure(s)
- Review of the homework
  - Self-monitoring
  - Notes from the previous session (optional)
  - Psychoeducational handout (optional)
  - Self-help book assignment (optional)
- Review of the CBT model
- Modification of the general CBT model to explain OCD
- Rationale for CBT for OCD
- Brief overview of the treatment
- Homework
  - Review of the rationale
  - New assignment
- Rapport and alliance building: Feedback, summary, and a take-home message

## MATERIALS NEEDED

- Self-report measure(s)
- Dry-erase board, easel, or clip board for you to use
- Clip board for the patient to take notes during the session
- Handouts/forms for homework (see Appendix B)
  - Self-Monitoring Forms (see Appendix B)
  - Self-help book recommendations (optional)

## CHECK ON SYMPTOMS

As was the case at the start of treatment Session 1, as well as all sessions going forward, you can have the patient provide three quick subjective ratings, using an average from 0 to 10, for (1) the severity of the OCD symptoms, (2) the amount of effort put into the treatment, and (3) the success the patient has had in managing the OCD symptoms since the last session. Ideally, these scores will be immediately added to a spreadsheet program (e.g., Microsoft Excel) and then charted (see the example for a patient who is four sessions into treatment in Figure 8.1; a blank form can be found in Appendix B, Form 6, Chart for Recording Check on OCD Symptoms) and graphed (see Figure 8.2) and shown to the patient for immediate feedback on how she is progressing in treatment. You and the patient can also examine the ratings together and look for connections between effort, success/control, and overall OCD symptom severity. In addition, depending on whether or not improvements are noted, you can either reinforce the patient for efforts made, normalize plateaus or slips in treatment, or problem-solve any stumbling blocks (e.g., motivation, insight, homework compliance, comorbidity issues, psychosocial stressor changes).

## Optional: Provide and Score Self–Report Measure(s)

As was the case at the start of treatment Session 1, as well as all sessions going forward, you can have the patient complete a brief, empirically based, self-report measure of OCD (e.g., OCI-R;

| Number | OCD Severity | Effort | Success/ Managing |
|--------|--------------|--------|-------------------|
| 1 | 9 | 3 | 1 |
| 2 | 9 | 5 | 2 |
| 3 | 8 | 7 | 4 |
| 4 | 7 | 8 | 5 |
| 5 | | | |
| 6 | | | |
| 7 | | | |
| 8 | | | |
| 9 | | | |
| 10 | | | |
| 11 | | | |
| 12 | | | |
| 13 | | | |
| 14 | | | |
| 15 | | | |
| 16 | | | |

**FIGURE 8.1.** Sample Chart for Recording Check on OCD Symptoms.

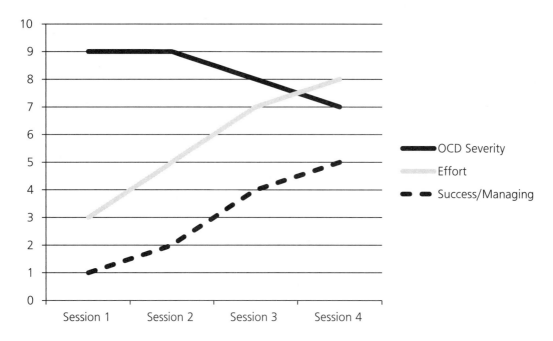

**FIGURE 8.2.** Sample graph of results of check on OCD symptoms.

available in Appendix C, Form 11) at the start of certain sessions as a more objective measure of treatment progress. It is advisable to have the patient complete it at a consistent time (e.g., just prior to the start of the session) and to score it at the start of the session, so that the patient can be given feedback on how the treatment is progressing. At this time, specific items representing particularly challenging situations/triggers may be identified, reviewed, and used to shape future in-session exposure exercises.

## REVIEW OF THE HOMEWORK

### Self-Monitoring

If the patient completed the self-monitoring assignment, be sure to reinforce him by offering praise and spending some time in the session reviewing several of the entries. This can help build rapport, increase motivation, and foster compliance with future assignments. Be sure to look for symptoms that the patient had not previously mentioned and ask the patient about them.

You can also provide corrective feedback on how to improve the monitoring, if necessary. For example, many patients with OCD have difficulty being succinct when completing an entry, and they often turn the monitoring forms into a personal journal or diary, writing in a narrative style. If this is the case, you can still reinforce the patient for making an effort, but then suggest that triggers are best described in a sentence or two and should be separated from obsessions, which in turn should be separated from rituals and the like. In this way, the patient can learn to be able to "see the cycle" as it is happening and be in a better place to stop it in the future.

If the patient failed to complete the assignment, you should consider spending some time asking the patient about what happened, reviewing the rationale for it, and problem-solving where necessary. You can then use the remainder of the time that was intended for the homework review to practice completing the monitoring form. You can use events that the patient recalls having occurred during the time between sessions and then collaborate with the patient to come up with a plan on how he will ensure that the monitoring is completed before the next session.

## Notes from the Previous Session (Optional)

If the patient took notes during the previous session and was asked to review them between sessions, be sure to ask whether she completed this task and, if so, reinforce her efforts by offering praise and spending some time in the session reviewing any questions or comments she has about them. If the patient failed to complete the assignment, you can spend some time asking her about what happened, reviewing the rationale for it, and problem-solving where necessary. You can then collaborate with the patient to come up with a plan on how she will ensure that the assignment will be completed before the next session.

## Psychoeducational Handout (Optional)

If the patient was given a psychoeducational handout on OCD (e.g., the NIH OCD Fact Sheet, available in Appendix B, Form 5) to review, be sure to ask whether he completed this task and, if so, reinforce the patient's efforts by offering praise and asking the patient for a shim ummary of the main points and any questions that arose while reviewing it. This will allow you to ensure that the patient has a solid understanding of the content before moving forward with the treatment. If the patient failed to complete the assignment, you can spend some time asking him about what happened, reviewing the rationale for it, and problem-solving where necessary. You can then collaborate with the patient to come up with a plan on how he will ensure that the assignment will be completed before the next session.

## Self-Help Book Assignment (Optional)

If the patient was assigned a self-help book (e.g., *Stop Obsessing!: How to Overcome Your Obsessions and Compulsions* by Edna Foa and Reid Wilson or *Overcoming Obsessive Thoughts: How to Gain Control of Your OCD* by Christine Purdon and David Clark), be sure to ask whether the patient was able to purchase it and if so, if she has started reading it. If the patient purchased the book and has started reading it, you can reinforce her efforts by offering praise and asking her for a summary of the main points and any questions that arose while reading it. This will allow you to ensure that the patient has a solid understanding of both the content of the book and how the book can be used to augment the treatment. If the patient failed to complete the assignment, you can spend some time asking her about what happened, reviewing the rationale for it, and problem-solving where necessary. You can then collaborate with the patient to come up with a plan on how she will ensure that the assignment will be completed before the next session.

## REVIEW OF THE CBT MODEL

You should review the general CBT model that was presented to the patient during the last session to ascertain how much information presented then the patient has absorbed. While attempting to make this discussion as interactive as possible, you should aim to cover the following points about the model: (1) it is based on a theory of psychological disorders that suggests that all situations can be broken down into three modalities we experience simultaneously: feelings, actions, and thoughts; (2) it places equal importance on each of these three modalities; (3) it asserts that each of the modalities connects with the other two; and (4) it suggests that if we learn to capitalize on the interconnections between thoughts, behaviors, and emotions, we can reduce emotional distress and attain a better quality of life by targeting maladaptive thoughts and problematic behaviors. You can then test the patient's understanding of the model by drawing out a blank CBT triangle on either a dry-erase board, flipchart, or notepad page and asking the patient to complete it, using as an example an upsetting situation he faced in the past week. Reinforce any effort the patient makes to explain the CBT triangle while also providing corrective feedback when necessary and asking if the patient has any questions before moving on.

## MODIFICATION OF THE GENERAL CBT MODEL TO EXPLAIN OCD

With the CBT triangle still in sight, you can now demonstrate to the patient how, with just some minor modifications, it is easy to see how OCD symptoms are triggered and maintained. Using either a different portion of the dry-erase board, flipchart, or new notepad page, you can "move" the word *situation* from the middle of the triangle to the top of the page and add the word *trigger* beside it. You can then move the word *thoughts* from one corner of the triangle to underneath the words *situation/trigger*, add the word *obsessions* beside it, and draw a bidirectional arrow from the situation/trigger to connect to the thoughts/obsessions (see Figure 8.3).

You can use this as an opportunity to (1) review the definition and key features of an obsession with the patient (e.g., unwanted, intrusive, repetitive, and distressing); and (2) introduce the idea to the patient that, while his OCD symptoms may seem to occur randomly and out of the blue, in fact, they frequently occur in highly predictable patterns (as likely was demonstrated in the self-monitoring that the patient completed for homework). Typically, they involve situations and triggers that have a special importance to the patient.

You can now emphasize the link between obsessions and anxiety by moving the word *feelings* from another corner of the CBT triangle, placing it underneath the words thoughts/obsessions, adding the word *anxiety* beside it and drawing a bidirectional arrow from the thoughts/obsessions to the feelings/anxiety (see Figure 8.4). You can also remind the patient that the connection between thoughts and feelings is bidirectional (i.e., that obsessions can generate anxiety and can also be generated when the patient feels anxious) and give some examples from the patient's intake evaluation (e.g., depending on the theme, it may be shaking hands [contamination], leaving home [harm/responsibility]). Sometimes patients will be highly aware of their obsessive thoughts but not the situations or triggers connected to them; at other times, they will report noticing only that certain situations or triggers make them anxious, without being able to report any awareness of specific obsessive thoughts. You can inform the patient that this is normal, particularly at the start of treatment, and you should encourage the patient to continue to use self-monitoring to become more aware of connections and patterns.

You can then move the word *actions* from the remaining corner of the triangle, place it underneath the words *feelings/anxiety*, add the words *rituals/compulsions* beside it, and draw a bidirec-

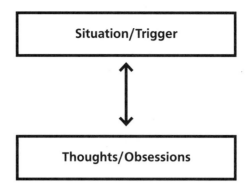

**FIGURE 8.3.** Beginning the CBT model of OCD.

tional arrow from the feelings/anxiety to the actions/rituals/compulsions (see Figure 8.5). You can use this as an opportunity to review the definition and key features of a ritual/compulsion with the patient (e.g., something the patient feels driven to do, in order to neutralize an obsession or trigger or feel less anxious). Be sure to emphasize that while many rituals are observable actions, they also can be performed as mental acts, and you should give some examples (e.g., thinking of a positive image if experiencing an intrusive image; counting to a certain number; mentally reviewing).

Note that some patients may ask why mental rituals would not be placed with the "thoughts/obsessions" part of the flowchart, as they represent a type of thought. You can point out that although mental rituals do indeed represent a type of thinking process, in terms of the CBT model of OCD they are best classified as (unobservable) actions because they represent something the patient feels compelled to do in order to feel less anxious or prevent a feared catastrophe from happening.

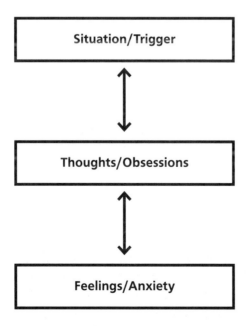

**FIGURE 8.4.** Continuing the CBT model of OCD.

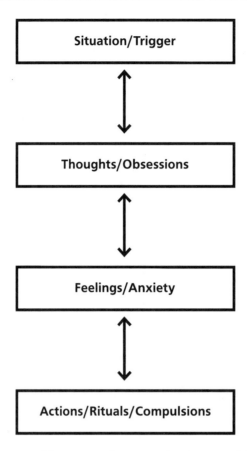

**FIGURE 8.5.** Adding compulsions to the CBT model of OCD.

You can then highlight the impact that performance of the actions/rituals/compulsions is intended to have on the anxiety (decrease it) and obsessions (neutralize them) by adding additional arrows to the model (see Figure 8.6) and then illustrate this point using several examples of both overt (observable) rituals and covert (mental) rituals that the patient reported during the intake evaluation. You can also note that, in terms of the CBT model of OCD, the patient's avoidance of situations/triggers and/or safety behaviors can also be placed in the actions/rituals/compulsions box (as these behaviors are also performed to help the patient feel less anxious and/or prevent a feared catastrophe from happening). You should provide several examples from the patient's intake evaluation.

Some patients may ask why the connection between the feelings/anxiety and the actions/rituals/compulsions is bidirectional. You can point out that while engaging in rituals/compulsions relieves anxiety in the short term, over time it also strengthens the connection between the rituals and the obsessions that caused the anxiety, such that engaging in a ritual can begin to trigger the very obsession and anxiety it was meant to neutralize. For example, many patients report that randomly engaging in a ritual (e.g., hand washing) often primes them to experience more obsessions. This can be illustrated by adding additional arrows to the model (see Figure 8.6).

Finally, you should note that the world may seem to be filled with an unlimited supply of situations and triggers: (1) not everyone diagnosed with OCD becomes anxious about the same things;

and (2) patients diagnosed with OCD are typically triggered by situations or objects that fit into certain themes. In addition, you can remind the patient that although almost everybody in the general population experiences the same unwanted, intrusive thoughts as individuals diagnosed with OCD, not everyone ends up with a diagnosis of OCD. As such, it is important to realize that one more step must exist in the model to allow it to explain why all people face the same triggers and can experience the same type of unwanted intrusive thoughts, but only certain people end up being diagnosed with OCD.

Explain to the patient that in order for an intrusive thought to be transformed into an obsession, it needs to be misinterpreted (i.e., misappraised) in a certain way (i.e., negatively) by the patient, which allows the intrusive thought to gain importance and, in turn, generate anxiety. This increase in importance also leads patients to pay more attention to the thoughts (and/or the triggers of the thoughts), which in turn causes patients to experience an increase in the number of triggers and/or frequency in the intrusive thoughts (i.e., it becomes an obsession—unwanted, intrusive, repetitive, and distressing).

In other words, you can explain that it is not actually the intrusive thoughts that generate the strong feelings of anxiety and distress and lead to the urges to ritualize, but rather what the patient *believes about* the intrusive thoughts. Provide the patient with several examples, based on information obtained during the intake evaluation or from the self-monitoring homework in order

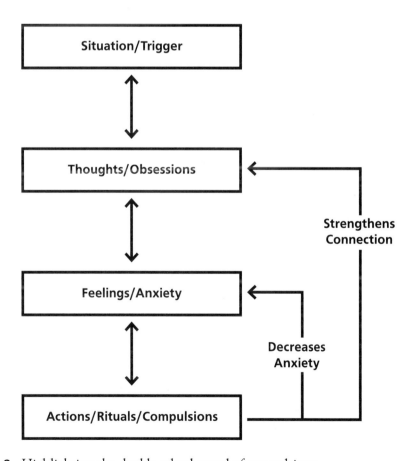

**FIGURE 8.6.** Highlighting the double-edged sword of compulsions.

to "customize" it to the patient and make sure that it "fits" with the patient's experience. Common categories of misappraisals include (1) overestimating the importance of thoughts, including a concept called thought–action fusion, (2) exhibiting an inflated sense of personal responsibility, (3) having an excessive need for certainty, (4) displaying an excessive need for control over thoughts, (5) overestimating threat, and (6) having an intolerance for the anxiety caused by the thoughts.

For example, patients with OCD may believe that they will be *responsible* for a burglary occurring if they fail to check to make sure a door is properly locked; or that having a thought about pushing an old woman into oncoming traffic means that they are *more likely* to actually do it (or is *just as bad* as having done it); or that they should be *in control* of the content of their thoughts at all times. You can illustrate the critical role of misappraisals in the CBT model of OCD by modifying it to include appraisals/interpretations between the thoughts/obsessions and the feelings/anxiety boxes (see Figure 8.7).

The above points will have greater impact if made in an engaging, conversational (vs. didactic) style. You can also get the patient to summarize the steps in the model or give the patient a "pop quiz" on the main points covered. At a minimum, be sure to frequently ask patients if they have any questions.

## RATIONALE FOR CBT FOR OCD

You should keep the diagram of the CBT model of OCD visible, so that it can be referenced while presenting the rationale for treatment. The rationale can include a discussion of the futility in trying to eliminate and/or avoid all potential OCD triggers in the world and a reminder of how attempting to avoid the triggers plays a key role in maintaining the disorder. You can also inform the patient of the equally futile task of trying to control or suppress unwanted thoughts and point out that making such an effort paradoxically causes an increase in the frequency and intensity of the thoughts (i.e., enhancement); even if the patient manages to successfully control the thoughts for a few moments, he frequently fights back all that much stronger (i.e., the rebound effect). Therapists commonly use an example to illustrate this notion, such as the "pink elephant" experiment (see the box on page 86). Next, you can remind the patient that anxiety is a normal and universal emotion, and even useful under the right circumstances, so unfortunately, we cannot eliminate it from the patient's life. Finally, you can point out that although the use of rituals may be an effective strategy for reducing anxiety in the short term, it does not appear to be an effective long-term strategy, as the patient's symptoms seem to have gotten worse over time and/or the patient would not need to seek treatment if this was the case.

Summarize the model by reminding the patient that while the use of avoidance and/or rituals may appear to have been an excellent way to reduce the anxiety caused by the various situations, triggers, and obsessive thoughts in the short term, this approach has failed as a long-term solution because the relief that the patient experienced made it seem like she had taken the right action to reduce the possibility of her feared outcome. You can explain that unfortunately, however, the patient's use of rituals has served to maintain the very OCD symptoms that she has been so desperate to be rid of because by using rituals she has never been able to test the accuracy of her beliefs about the situations, triggers, and obsessive thoughts or to build any confidence in her abil-

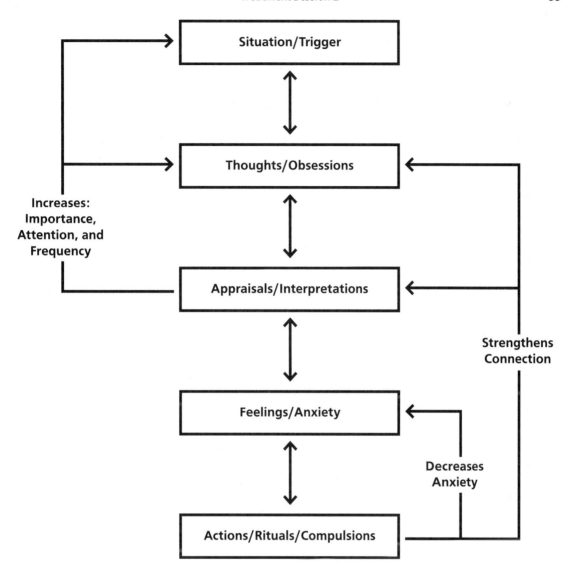

**FIGURE 8.7.** Completing the CBT model of OCD by adding the role of appraisals/interpretations.

ity to manage her anxiety without using them—which has given them more power in the long term. You can explain that, unless the patient is willing to directly confront the feared situation, trigger, obsessive thought, or the anxiety itself, she will never be able to find out if the consequence that she fears so much will actually occur. As a result, the anxiety will return in similar situations, which will force the patient to continue to rely on the use of her rituals with more and more frequency and intensity.

You can explain that, given how poorly avoidance and ritualizing work in the long term, the primary goal of the treatment is simply to have the patient gradually, systematically, and repeatedly face the various situations, triggers, and obsessive thoughts he fears, without doing any of the things he has typically done to try to mitigate them (i.e., rituals or avoidance). You can explain to the patient that in so doing, he will finally have the chance to test out his beliefs, which will

---

### The Pink Elephant Experiment

THERAPIST: As you can see by the model we just drew to explain your OCD cycle, trying to control or suppress your unwanted thoughts only seems to have made them increase in frequency and feel even more intense. In addition, you noted that on those rare occasions where you have mustered all of your strength and energy and have somehow succeeded in pushing aside your unwanted thoughts for a few moments, they often seem to have come rushing back in all that much stronger, just when you believed you could finally let your guard down. Why do you think this is the case?

PATIENT: Exactly. I don't know. It's so draining to watch out for the thoughts and triggers and to be ready to fight them all the time, and yet, despite my best efforts, it seems like I am slowly losing the battle.

THERAPIST: That sounds really exhausting and frustrating.

PATIENT: Exactly. But what else am I supposed to do?

THERAPIST: Well, I am wondering if you see any connection between your effort to fight the thoughts and the fact that they are coming back so often?

PATIENT: Yes. As I just said, it seems like I have to fight them all the time, because they keep coming back.

THERAPIST: I know that seems a little backward, but did you ever consider that it is because you are fighting so hard against them, that they keep coming back stronger and stronger, instead of the other way around?

PATIENT: Huh? I don't see the difference.

THERAPIST: Well, perhaps doing a little thought experiment might help. First, close your eyes. Now, imagine a pink elephant as vividly as you can. It has big pink floppy ears, and a big pink trunk, and a little pink tail. And when I say pink, I mean hot pink! Can you picture it? What does it look like: cartoon elephant or a real elephant that you would see in the zoo?

PATIENT: OK. I can picture it. It looks like a bright pink version of Dumbo!

THERAPIST: Excellent. Now, for the next few minutes, I want you to try your absolute hardest to *not* think about pink Dumbo. Put all of your effort into thinking about *anything else* but pink Dumbo. Imagine your life depended on you *not* thinking of Pink Dumbo.

PATIENT: OK. I'll try.

THERAPIST: Excellent. Please let me know when you've successfully rid yourself of any thoughts of pink Dumbo.

PATIENT: Hey! I can't seem to stop thinking of him!

THERAPIST: Interesting, huh? What do you make of the experiment?

---

help him break the link between the various triggers and thoughts and his feelings of anxiety (i.e., change the way you think, and you can change the way you feel). You can explain to the patient that, though scary, this is the only way he will ever be able to learn anything new about his symptoms and if he is unwilling to change how he thinks and acts, he will likely continue to experience the same feelings.

You can inform the patient that changing how he thinks and acts can be accomplished in two main ways: (1) breaking the link between using avoidance and/or rituals to manage his feelings of anxiety by having him engage in Ex/RP and (2) breaking the link between experiencing an obsessive thought and feeling anxious by having him learn to develop a new relationship with his thoughts through various cognitive exercises (including cognitive restructuring, metacognitive techniques, and acceptance and commitment therapy strategies) in order to learn to reappraise what his thoughts are really all about.

First, you can explain the role of habituation in the exposure process. You can note how the research has shown that when people face the things (e.g., situations, triggers, and thoughts) they fear and maintain contact with these feared things for a long enough period of time, their anxiety eventually declines. You can inform the patient that this is what is meant by the term *exposure*. You may add that if exposure is set up in a hierarchical (i.e., stepwise) manner and systematically, the patient's anxiety should decrease not only *within* each exposure exercise, but also *between* each exposure trial, leading to less and less anticipatory anxiety with each subsequent exercise, until eventually the situations, triggers, and obsessive thoughts will no longer generate much anxiety at all. Emphasize that this is something that the patient will *feel* as he moves through the treatment, which will give him more confidence in the treatment and more motivation to continue up the hierarchy. This process can be illustrated using a graph of habituation (see Figure 8.8).

Next, you can emphasize the importance of using the technique of exposure not just to facilitate the process of habituation, but also to create a context for new learning to occur—be it about the situations, triggers, obsessive thoughts, or anxiety, as doing so will maximize the benefits of the treatment. You can explain that patients with problematic beliefs are more successful at restructuring their beliefs when they are willing to experience the emotions attached to their beliefs, and this is most easily accomplished by having patients face their fears (i.e., engage in exposure). In other words, in order for the patient to learn how to challenge her beliefs about the OCD symptoms, the anxiety that they cause, the feared consequences, and the importance of her rituals, she will need to create opportunities (e.g., via exposure exercises) for her feelings

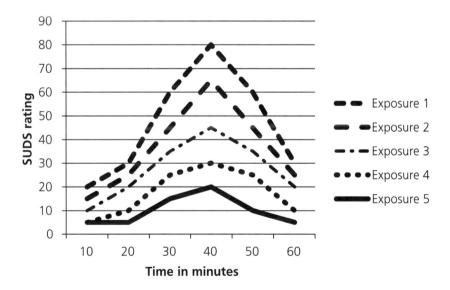

**FIGURE 8.8.** Sample graph of habituation.

and thoughts to be *activated*, and then she will have to *test her beliefs* in various ways, such as through the use of ritual prevention (e.g., she can learn that anxiety decreases without needing to resort to rituals) or hypothesis testing (e.g., she can learn that it is not the ritualizing that prevents harm to the patient or someone else she cares about by creating an experiment in which this hypothesis is tested in session). Either way, this new learning helps maximize the benefits of exposure and, when paired with the process of habituation, makes it easier to resist performing the rituals in the future.

At this point, you can emphasize that exposure is never conducted by surprise and never against the patient's will. In fact, you can remind the patient of the CBT principle of *collaborative empiricism* and observe that the two of you will need to form a scientific *team* that will work together to examine and test out the patient's beliefs about his OCD symptoms, the anxiety that they cause, and the importance of rituals. This will involve creating experiments (i.e., exposure exercises) to be performed together in session, so that the patient can learn how to become his own cognitive behavior therapist and conduct the same types of experiments on his own—at first between sessions and then eventually once the treatment has ended. You can also stress that the therapy will be challenging at first as, much like learning any new skill, it takes a lot of time and effort to practice, but it will get easier in time.

Inform the patient that the treatment will begin by focusing on the aspect of the model that is easier to control: the need to perform rituals. In particular, in keeping with the principle of collaborative empiricism, the two of you will begin to set up a series of experiments that will aim to test out two beliefs thought to be responsible for fueling the OCD cycle: (1) that unless situations, triggers, obsessive thoughts, and anxiety are avoided or managed using rituals, the patient's anxiety will either spiral out of control, never coming down on its own, or the patient will go crazy; and (2) that performing rituals actually prevents something bad from happening to the patient or some other important person in his life (e.g., a loved one, coworker, neighbor). You can inform the patient that if he can learn something new about these two beliefs (e.g., that they are inaccurate), then the situations, triggers, obsessive thoughts, and anxiety will become less important, resulting in less attention being paid to them, and ultimately, causing them to appear less frequently.

Inform the patient that the treatment will also teach her to develop a new relationship with her thoughts. You can inform her that this will be done by teaching her how to reappraise the *meaning behind the thoughts* in a more accurate and rational manner and, in so doing, break the connection between experiencing an obsessive thought and feeling anxious about it. Tell the patient that there are many ways to accomplish this goal, including (1) learning to accept, tolerate, and mindfully observe intrusive thoughts; (2) increasing awareness of the misappraisals that are linked to the intrusive thoughts and generating alternatives to the misappraisals that contribute to her anxiety; (3) gathering evidence for and against the misappraisals and alternatives; (4) setting up experiments to directly test any predictions made based on her appraisals and assumptions about the unwanted intrusive thoughts; and (5) learning to "defuse" or disentangle herself from her thoughts. Ultimately, all of the methods listed above have a single aim: to teach the patient to be a *more flexible thinker*.

Recall that cognitive techniques are designed to target the patient's *appraisals* of the thoughts and *not* the *obsessive thoughts* per se. As such, you must be sure to *identify the appraisal behind the obsessive thought* before commencing with this portion of the therapy. It is also important that you do *not* use cognitive techniques to try to *disconfirm* the patient's appraisals and beliefs, but rather help the patient to generate *alternative* appraisals and consider the evidence for and against these alternative appraisals, and in so doing, learn to tolerate uncertainty. Although newer approaches (e.g., mindfulness, acceptance and commitment therapy) can be applied to the thoughts directly, they still do not attempt to challenge or change the thoughts. Instead they aim to help the patient develop a new relationship with the thoughts.

For example, a patient with OCD may report that he performs checking rituals (e.g., checking to make sure relatives are alive and well) that are triggered when he has to go to work or has not heard from them in some time). Upon some investigation, you may discover that that the checking rituals are in response to the obsessive thought, "Something bad could have happened to them!" Trying to challenge the thought at this level (e.g., helping the patient dispute the idea that any-thing bad could have happened), however, will indirectly teach the patient that this thought must be important (why else would my therapist focus on it), encourage the patient to seek certainty in a situation where there can be no certainty (bad things can happen at any time), and also fail to help the patient modify the appraisal that is making the thought so anxiety provoking (e.g., intolerance of uncertainty, importance of thoughts, inflated responsibility).

By identifying the appraisal(s) behind the obsessive thoughts, you and the patient can then scrutinize the accuracy of the appraisal and/or set up an appropriate behavioral experiment to test it out. For example, a patient experiencing obsessive thoughts that something bad could happen to his relatives may appraise this experience to mean that having the thought indicates it is impor-tant, and therefore, if he does not check on their well-being, he will be responsible if something bad happens to them. Rather than targeting the *content* of the obsession, you and the patient can use cognitive techniques to challenge the *appraisal* that all thoughts are important along with the inflated responsibility the patient is experiencing—all while either conducting a behavioral experiment designed to increase the patient's tolerance of uncertainty (e.g., withhold a check-in with a specific family member and predict a specific negative outcome) or engaging in Ex/RP (e.g., imagining something bad happening to a family member and not checking in).

By using cognitive strategies (see Chapter 14) to modify the appraisal and decrease its strength, the patient should experience less anxiety at the thought that something bad could happen to his relatives, which would make it easier for him to engage in behavioral experiments and/or ritual prevention. This in turn allows the patient to reconsider the role his rituals play in keeping his relatives safe. Finally, as the strength of the patient's belief in the appraisal decreases, the importance the patient gives to the thoughts and triggers should also decrease, which would decrease the attention he pays to the triggers and thoughts and lead to a perceived decrease in their frequency.

Emphasize tht it is important that the patient understand and agree with the CBT model of OCD and the rationale for treatment or else it is unlikely that the two of you will have success. Ask if the patient has any questions or concerns and be sure to clarify any misunderstandings or misconceptions before moving on to overview of the treatment.

## BRIEF OVERVIEW OF THE TREATMENT

Inform the patient that in the next session, the agenda will focus on collaborating to generate a "master list" of all of the various situations, triggers, and obsessive thoughts that make the patient anxious. Explain that once this master list is generated, the two of you will then collaborate on making a scale to rate the degree of anxiety that the items on the master list generate, from 0 to 10 (where 0 would represent no anxiety and 10 would represent the maximum anxiety).

Explain to the patient that once each of the items is rated, they will then be rank ordered from lowest to highest and that this list of rank-ordered items (i.e., hierarchy) will then be used as the "backbone" for the treatment. You can forewarn the patient that, beginning the visit after the next, the treatment will involve exposing him to the situations, triggers, and obsessive thoughts that he has previously worked so hard to avoid, suppress, and/or neutralize in some way, and preventing the rituals that he has used to feel better in the short term (i.e., Ex/RP).

The Ex/RP will be conducted in collaboration with the patient and will start with the items from the master list that fall in the low–moderate anxiety range. You can inform the patient that each exposure trial will be planned in advance and will be highly structured. In addition, whenever possible, the two of you will initially conduct each exposure trial together in your sessions, and then collaborate on designing a logical extension of the work done in session for the patient to work on between sessions for homework.

Be sure to warn the patient that if the two of you are doing things correctly, she should feel anxious for a while. Inform the patient that this is the natural short-term price she must pay for having avoided exposing herself to situations, triggers, and obsessive thoughts for so long. Add, however, that the anxiety she initially feels in the short term should gradually decline as she spends more and more time facing her fears and questioning her assumptions related to the situations, triggers, and obsessive thoughts that cause them, rather than engaging in rituals to manage them. Ultimately, this will help her to break the link between using a ritual and feeling less anxious and help her to develop a new relationship with her thoughts in the long term.

Emphasize that the treatment is intense and requires the patient to devote a great deal of time and effort to practicing the skills being taught to maximize the outcome. If the treatment allows for phone sessions between the office visits, remind the patient of how and when they will be utilized—including to offer the patient support (not reassurance) in managing the task of Ex/RP. You should also warn the patient that if she is not willing to practice the skills each and every day, she will likely not benefit from the treatment and you should use this discussion to transition to the topic of homework for the week.

# HOMEWORK

## Review of the Rationale

Review the analogy of learning OCD skills being like learning a new language, musical instrument, or sport. Namely, it takes more than a once-weekly, hour-long office visit to become proficient at it. You should add that, in this case, the patient may not only have to learn a new approach, but also unlearn "bad habits" she has developed to help manage the OCD. Warn the patient that this can often make the task even more challenging—like having to unlearn a bad golf swing!

Review the strong connection between homework compliance and treatment outcome and remind the patient that he will be learning to test out ideas that the two of you generate in session to see how well they work in the "real world" outside your office. Be sure to emphasize that the data the patient collects between sessions will be used to shape the case formulation and treatment plan; the treatment is designed to be flexible so that you can do more of the things that are benefiting the patient and less of the things that are not. Note that without between-session data, these adjustments may not be made as quickly or as efficiently, if at all, and the treatment may not be as effective.

Remind the patient that it is normal for patients to struggle with completing the homework at times. The assignments call on patients to take a "leap of faith" that the results generated in the session will be the same as the results produced outside of sessions. In addition, many patients struggle to complete exercises without the aid and guidance of the therapist. You should remind that patient that some steps can be taken to maximize the chances of success, including (1) being clear on how each exercise is connected to their broader treatment goal(s), (2) understanding what exactly needs to be done, how, when and where to do it, for how long, and how to record it, (3) anticipating any potential roadblocks in getting it done and problem-solving in advance how to overcome them, and (4) starting small.

For patients who have elected to enlist the help of a family member or friend as a coach in order to complete the homework, you should check to see how this worked out and ideally, save a few minutes to check in with the coach as well. If necessary, reeducate the coach about how best to help (e.g., encourage, remind, and give support vs. coerce or give reassurance) in order to maximize the benefits and minimize the costs of using a coach. If you will be acting as coach to the patient between sessions (i.e., offering phone support sessions), remind the patient about the rules (e.g., frequency, length, and format) of the sessions and confirm the next coaching session.

## New Assignment

As it is still early in the treatment, it is wise to have the patient once again review the notes taken—during both this session and the previous one—and return with a summary and any questions. It can also be useful to provide the patient with a copy of the CBT model of OCD that was introduced this session (see Appendix B, Form 7). In addition, you can ask the patient to continue to self-monitor the OCD symptoms, paying attention to patterns and new symptoms that may emerge. You can also remind the patient of any corrections that should made based on what was observed when reviewing the self-monitoring assignment from last week at the beginning of the session. Finally, if a self-help book was assigned to augment the treatment, the patient can be asked to either start or continue reading it.

As was the case after assigning the homework at the end of Session 1, you should check to make sure that the patient agrees on the usefulness of the assignments and connection to the broader goals of treatment. If the patient agrees on the usefulness of the assignment and can see the connection to the broader goals of treatment, you can then check to make sure the patient has enough copies of the Self-Monitoring Form (see Figure 7.3 and Appendix B, Form 4) and plan when and where self-monitoring will be done.

If the patient does not agree that this would be a useful assignment and/or cannot connect it to the broader treatment goal(s), you can address these issues before moving ahead. Sometimes a review of the rationale or model will help. At other times a modification of the task may increase the patient's willingness to try it. In any event, the patient's resistance should be discussed and addressed before moving ahead; simply insisting that the patient complete the assignment will not likely be effective and would violate the collaborative nature of the treatment.

# RAPPORT AND ALLIANCE BUILDING: FEEDBACK, SUMMARY, AND TAKE-HOME MESSAGE

Finally, be sure to continue to build rapport, trust, and a strong working alliance with the patient by eliciting feedback about what he liked and disliked about the session and the way it was managed. In this case, it can be helpful to elicit feedback from the patient on what you have presented in terms of the OCD models, the rationale for treatment, and the second homework assignment. You can also *give* feedback to the patient about anything positive that you noticed (during the session, between the sessions, since the initial intake, etc.) as well as provide constructive, corrective feedback if necessary. You and the patient can also take turns (ideally having the patient start) at summarizing the main points of the session, presenting a succinct summary of the highlights of what was done. Based on this collaborative summary, you can ask the patient for a take-home message (i.e., a key principle, theme, or lesson) with which he will leave the session and approach the world (e.g., "Based on what was covered this week, what's different about how you view your OCD or even the world?").

---

### TAKE-HOME MESSAGE FROM TREATMENT SESSION 2

Treatment Session 2 builds on the foundation started in treatment Session 1 by reviewing the CBT model and then expanding it to account for OCD. This CBT model of OCD is then used to explain how the patient's OCD is being maintained and how it can be treated. By presenting more detailed, specific information to the patient, you will have the opportunity once again to instill hope in the patient and boost the patient's confidence in both you and the treatment. In addition, this session sets the stage for what lies ahead in the treatment and presents an overview of what patients can expect in terms of both structure and process. This can go a long way toward enhancing the patient's motivation and commitment to the treatment when facing challenging items on the hierarchy. The assignment of the monitoring and review of session notes allows you to ascertain the patient's level of the motivation, insight, and comprehension. The information obtained from the monitoring can be used as a baseline measure of OCD symptom severity, as well as a way to generate items for the hierarchy construction at Session 3. Finally, rapport, trust, and alliance can continue to be built through soliciting and providing feedback, as well as through agreeing on a summary of the session and a take-home message for the patient.

---

# CHAPTER 9

# Treatment Session 3

## SESSION COMPONENTS

- Check on symptoms
  - Optional: Provide and score self-report measure(s)
- Review of the homework
  - Self-monitoring
  - Notes from the previous session (optional)
  - Psychoeducational handouts (optional)
    - CBT model of OCD
    - NIH Fact Sheet on Obsessive–Compulsive Disorder
  - Self-help book assignment (optional)
- Review of the CBT model of OCD
- Review rationale for CBT for OCD
- Explain the concept of SUDS and create a personalized scale
- Generate items for the exposure hierarchy
- Homework
  - Review of the rationale
  - New assignments
- Rapport and alliance building: Feedback, summary, and a take-home message

## MATERIALS NEEDED

- Self-report measure(s)
- Dry-erase board, easel, or clip board for you to use
- Clip board for the patient to take notes during the session
- Hierarchy Construction Worksheet
- Handouts/forms for homework (see Appendix B)
  - Self-Monitoring Forms (see Appendix B)
  - Copy of master list of hierarchy items with SUDS ratings
  - Materials needed for first exposure (if any)
  - Self-help book recommendations (optional)

# CHECK ON SYMPTOMS

As was the case at the start of the previous two sessions, be sure to have the patient do a brief self-assessment, using an average from 0 to 10, of (1) the severity of the OCD symptoms, (2) the amount of effort she put into the treatment, and (3) the success she has had in managing the OCD symptoms since the last session. Ideally, you will once again immediately chart these scores (see Appendix B, Form 6) and then add them to a spreadsheet program, graph the scores, and then show them to the patient so that she can receive immediate feedback on how the treatment is progressing. You and the patient can examine the ratings together and look for connections between effort, success/control, and overall OCD symptom severity. In addition, depending on whether or not improvements are noted, you can either reinforce the patient for efforts made, normalize plateaus or slips in treatment, or problem-solve any stumbling blocks with her (e.g., motivation, insight, homework compliance, comorbidity issues, psychosocial stressor changes).

## Optional: Provide and Score Self-Report Measure(s)

As mentioned at the start of treatment Session 2, it can be useful and informative to have the patient complete a brief, empirically based, self-report measure of OCD (e.g., the OCI-R; see Appendix C, Form 11) at the start of certain sessions (e.g., weekly, monthly) to have a more objective measure of how treatment is progressing. As a reminder, if using this form, it is advisable to have the patient complete it at a consistent time (e.g., just prior to the start of the session) and to score it at the start of the session. The patient can therefore be given immediate feedback on how treatment is progressing in general, as well as on any specific items that may be reviewed and used to shape future in-session exposure exercises,

# REVIEW OF THE HOMEWORK

## Self-Monitoring

As was the case in treatment Session 2, if the patient completed the self-monitoring assignment, you can reinforce him by offering praise and spending some time in the session reviewing several of the entries on the Self-Monitoring Form (Appendix B, Form 4). You can look for symptoms that the patient had not previously mentioned and ask him about them, and you can also offer continued feedback on how he can improve the monitoring, if necessary. You can also ask the patient if any rituals were left off the monitoring form.

For example, some patients may stop recording rituals that they had recorded the previous week, even though they still experienced them between sessions, thinking that you already know about them. If this is the case, you and the patient can decide as a team what the best course of action is going forward: to record all rituals no matter what (which gives the most accurate look at how much the OCD has been impacting the patient's life in the past week and incentivizes the patient to prevent ritualizing so that he doesn't have to write them, but it can be cumbersome and time consuming) versus only recording new rituals (which is less time consuming for the patient and allows new rituals to be accommodated into the treatment plan, but gives a less accurate overall picture of the impact) versus some other arrangement (e.g., recording new rituals and new triggers of old rituals). Often the decision is best made if the *function* of the homework assignment (which can change from week to week) is made clear. Thus, you and the patient should decide what "data" the assignment is intended to generate and how this data will be used to inform the treatment. Then the homework can be designed in a way that allows the necessary data to be collected without overburdening the patient (or yourself).

If the patient failed to complete the assignment, you can spend some time asking him about what happened (with different lines of questioning depending on whether the patient had completed the assignment the week before), reviewing the rationale for it, and problem solving where necessary (e.g., consider making the monitoring easier if the patient has failed to complete it for two weeks in a row). You can then use the remainder of the time that was intended for the homework review to practice completing the Self-Monitoring Form (see Appendix B, Form 4), using events that the patient recalls having occurred during the time between sessions, and then collaborate with him to come up with a plan on how he will ensure that the monitoring is completed before the next session.

## Notes from the Previous Session (Optional)

If the patient took notes during the previous session and was asked to review the notes between sessions for homework, be sure to ask whether she completed this task and, if so, reinforce her efforts by offering praise and reviewing any questions or comments she has about them. If the patient failed to complete the assignment, you can spend some time asking her about what happened, reviewing the rationale for it, and problem-solving where necessary. You can then collaborate with the patient to come up with a plan on how she will ensure that the assignment will be completed before the next session.

## Psychoeducational Handouts (Optional)

If the patient was given psychoeducational handouts (e.g., the CBT model of OCD, NIH Fact Sheet on Obsessive–Compulsive Disorder) to review for homework, be sure to ask whether he completed this task and, if so, reinforce his efforts by offering praise and either asking him for a summary of the main points or answering any questions or comments he has about them. If the patient failed to complete this assignment, you can spend some time asking him about what seems to have interfered with it getting accomplished, reviewing the rationale for it, and problem-solving where necessary (e.g., was it a motivational issue, an outside distractor, too challenging, not useful, not clear?). You can then collaborate with the patient to determine whether the assignment is worth repeating and, if so, come up with a plan on how it will be completed before the next session.

## Self-Help Book Assignment (Optional)

If the patient was assigned a self-help book (e.g., *Stop Obsessing!: How to Overcome Your Obsessions and Compulsions* by Edna Foa and Reid Wilson and/or *Overcoming Obsessive Thoughts: How to Gain Control of Your OCD* by Christine Purdon and David A. Clark, see Appendix A) and had already started reading it the previous week, you can reinforce her efforts by offering praise and asking her for a summary of the main points and any questions that arose while she was reading it. Ensure that the patient's understanding of the content is sound and lines up with the treatment plan before moving on.

If the patient failed to complete the assignment, you can spend some time inquiring about what happened (especially if he has now failed to start the assignment twice), reviewing the rationale for using a self-help book to augment the therapy, and helping him to identify and problem-solve roadblocks, if necessary. Finally, you should collaborate with the patient to determine whether the assignment is worth repeating and, if so, come up with a plan on how it will be completed before the next session.

## REVIEW OF THE CBT MODEL OF OCD

Be sure to review the CBT model of OCD that you presented to the patient in the previous session in order to ascertain how much of the information she has absorbed. If you gave the patient a copy of the CBT model of OCD to examine for homework and reviewed the model during the review of homework phase of this session (see above), then you can skip to the review of the rationale for CBT for OCD in the next section (see below). If not, you can ask if the patient has any questions about the CBT model of OCD and answer them thoroughly before moving on. If the patient does not have any questions, you can assess how well he understands the model by either quizzing him on it or having him present the model (e.g., in a reverse role play or by asking the patient to draw the CBT model of OCD using an example from his week).

No matter the format, you should aim to be Socratic rather than didactic during the review, in order to make this discussion as interactive as possible. The review can include the following points about the model: (1) it shows how obsessions (thoughts) and compulsions (actions as well as thoughts) are linked through anxiety; (2) it shows how compulsions may decrease anxiety in the short term by neutralizing thoughts and triggers, but over time it also strengthens the connection between needing to ritualize when experiencing an obsession or feeling anxious; (3) for an intrusive thought to become an obsession, it needs to be misinterpreted by the patient; and (4) this misinterpretation or misappraisal gives the thought more importance, which leads the patient to pay more attention to it and thus notice it with greater frequency. Reinforce the patient for making an effort to try this, while also providing corrective feedback when necessary, and before moving on be sure to ask if the patient has any questions.

## REVIEW RATIONALE FOR CBT FOR OCD

Ask the patient if she has any questions about how the treatment will work and answer them thoroughly before moving on. If the patient does not have any questions about the rationale for CBT for OCD, you can assess how well the patient understands the rationale by either quizzing her on it or having her present it to you (e.g., in a reverse role-play).

The review can include the following points about the rationale: (1) anxiety is a normal and universal emotion, and even useful under the right circumstances, so unfortunately, it cannot be eliminated, (2) attempting to control triggers and thoughts through avoidance, suppression, or rituals may work in the short term but (3) these strategies only make things worse in the long term because they prevent the patient from testing the accuracy of her beliefs about the situations, triggers, obsessive thoughts, and emotions. As a result, the primary goal of the treatment is to have the patient *gradually, systematically, and repeatedly* face the various situations, triggers, and obsessive thoughts that she fears (i.e., engage in exposure), (1) without doing any of the things she typically does to try to feel better (i.e., engage in ritual prevention) and (2) with the intention of learning to reappraise her thoughts so that she can develop a new relationship with them. In so doing, patients are able to (1) break the connection between using avoidance and rituals to feel less anxious and (2) break the link between experiencing an obsessive thought and feeling anxious.

## EXPLAIN THE CONCEPT OF SUDS AND CREATE A PERSONALIZED SCALE

Explain to the patient that everybody experiences anxiety at times, but what makes one person anxious may not have the same effect on another person; therefore, just *how* anxious different people get when confronting the same trigger is highly *subjective*. To illustrate this point, you can use as an example watching a scary movie in a theater: some people will scream out loud and cover their eyes at certain parts, whereas other people watching the same scene will not feel scared at all, and still others will feel mildly anxious but not to the point of screaming or turning away.

Explain to the patient that, unfortunately, unlike other areas of medicine that can assess illnesses by using blood tests to examine the levels of certain markers in the blood, there are no easy tests available for measuring her level of anxiety. As a result, in the same way that the "Faces" scale is used to help patients describe their level of pain to their doctors or dentists, in CBT we have created a subjective rating scale to help patients describe their level of distress (i.e., anxiety) to their therapists. This is called the Subjective Units of Distress Scale (SUDS).

Inform the patient that in the case of OCD, the SUDS allows you to measure each patient's subjective reaction to various situations, triggers, and obsessive thoughts in concrete numbers. You can explain that the scale range is typically set from 0 to 10 (although some patients may prefer to use a 0–100 scale) and that a rating of 0 is meant to represent a time in which the patient is not anxious at all, whereas a rating of 10 (or 100) is meant to represent a time in which the patient is extremely anxious, often to the point of experiencing panic-like symptoms or even full-scale panic attacks. You can ask which scale the patient would prefer to use: 0–10 or 0–100. (Note: if using 0–100, do not allow values of less than 5 points.)

You can also have the patient "anchor" the scale by linking real experiences from her life, ideally those that are fairly recent and unrelated to her OCD symptoms, to the 0, 5, and 10 values. You should consider giving the patient a handout with a picture of the scale on it to help fill in anchor points as you create them (see Figure 9.1 for a sample SUDS and Appendix B, Form 8, for a SUDS template). For example, you might ask the patient to recall a specific time in the past year when she was either not experiencing any anxiety or only very slight anxiety or (for chronically anxious patients) the least anxiety. You can have the patient describe the time in some detail and then "anchor" this event to the score of 0 on the patient's SUDS. It is important to try to get a *specific scenario*, so that it will be easy for the patient to recall and make comparisons with the scenario when generating items for the exposure hierarchy later in treatment. In much the same

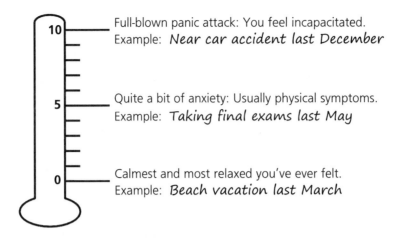

**FIGURE 9.1.** Sample SUDS template.

way, you can repeat the process for anchoring the *highest* end of the scale, and finally, the *middle* of the scale.

Finally, be sure to link the SUDS to the treatment rationale (see the previous section) by reminding the patient that because Ex/RP involves the systematic, prolonged, and repeated exposure to situations, triggers, and obsessive thoughts that cause anxiety, having a SUDS will allow the two of you to rank-order the patient's triggers from lowest to highest, so that the treatment can begin by having the patient confront some of the (relatively) less anxiety-provoking triggers and then gradually work toward confronting some of the more challenging triggers. You should ensure that the patient grasps the concept of SUDS by having her practice using the scale during the session for a few of her known triggers. You can find a handout—Subjective Units of Distress Scale (SUDS)—to give to patients on the concept of SUDS in Appendix B, Form 8.

## GENERATE ITEMS FOR THE EXPOSURE HIERARCHY

Explain that the goal now is to generate a master list of all the situations, triggers, and obsessive thoughts that have been making the patient anxious and/or are being avoided, and then to rate each one using the patient's SUDS in order to estimate how much anxiety each item would generate if encountered today. These items will then be ranked from lowest to highest, based on the SUDS ratings. You can note that, instead of trying to get all of the items in the proper order now, this should be treated like a brainstorming phase, with the final ordering of the items to be determined afterward and presented to the patient for approval. Inform the patient that once the hierarchy has been approved, it will be used as the foundation for the remainder of the treatment sessions (while allowing for new items to be added to it if they are discovered along the way).

If the patient has been compliant in completing the self-monitoring homework, you can reinforce this by using the situations, triggers, and thoughts that were monitored as a starting point for the hierarchy construction. If the patient has not been compliant with the homework or as a supplement to the homework, you can also start the hierarchy construction process by using any of the empirically based measures (e.g., Y-BOCS symptom checklist) that were administered, and/

or information that was gathered, during the intake. Regardless of the method used, be sure to ask the patient for any additional situations, triggers, and obsessive thoughts that she fears, starting with external situations and triggers (as these tend to be the easiest for patients to recall and report) and then moving on to anxiety-provoking thoughts, images, and body sensations.

While generating items for the hierarchy, it is also useful to inquire about and note any rituals and other safety behaviors that the patient engages in; at some point in the treatment, it will be important to ensure that the patient engages in the exposure exercises without using any of them. If necessary, this can be accomplished in a graduated way by conducting experiments on the outcome of the exposure exercises with and without their use. It is therefore important for you to gather information about the patient's feared *consequences* of the obsessions and/or experiencing of anxiety, for it is these beliefs that will need to be tested during the exposure exercises—with and without safety behaviors. This will ensure that the exposure exercises enhance the process of habitation as well as allow for new learning to occur.

After generating a master list of the situations, triggers, and obsessive thoughts that cause the patient to become anxious and getting a SUDS rating for each, you can then rank-order the list from highest to lowest SUDS. With this task in mind, it can be helpful to enter all of the items and their respective SUDS ratings in an electronic spreadsheet (e.g., Microsoft Excel), which then allows for items to be sorted from highest to lowest SUDS rating with just a click of the mouse. In addition, new items can then be added into the spreadsheet as they are discovered, and items currently in the spreadsheet can be edited or deleted as needed. New columns can also be added with ease, when reassessing SUDS at different points in the treatment. If it is too cumbersome to enter right into Excel during the session, you can use a copy of the Hierarchy Construction Worksheet (see Appendix B, Form 9) during the session and then enter the information into Excel between sessions.

A common issue that therapists face is whether patients with symptoms fitting multiple OCD categories should have several separate hierarchies or one mixed hierarchy. For example, you may wonder whether you should construct two separate hierarchies for a patient who has both washing and checking rituals or simply construct one hierarchy that includes both categories of rituals. Most typically, therapists tend to generate a single hierarchy, with items included from *all* categories, which are ranked by SUDS ratings. This way, the patient learns to confront all aspects of the OCD simultaneously, while still benefiting from a hierarchical approach.

Another common issue that therapists face involves deciding on how many items to include in the final hierarchy. Although the research literature has not adequately addressed this issue, several practical issues can be considered when determining the ideal number of items for the hierarchy. These include the fact that (1) the therapy is time-limited; (2) there should be a range of items to allow for maximum generalization of the treatment into the "real world" of the patient; (3) there should be enough items to allow for a range of SUDS ratings, so the patient can proceed in small steps; (4) the items need to be able to generate at least moderate anxiety for optimal exposure and habituation to occur; (5) the items need to be able to create the context for new learning to occur; (6) the items may shift in SUDS ranking as the patient works up the hierarchy; and (7) the goal is to get to the most anxiety-provoking items as quickly as possible in the treatment.

As a result, it may be best for you to generate and keep a "master list" of many items, while coming to an agreement with the patient about how many (and which) items will be *focused on* during the exposure sessions and which will be *assigned for homework and only practiced in session if necessary.* For example, an ideal hierarchy would contain items representing the range of SUDS ratings from 0 to 10, with perhaps one or two different items at each level. The in-session exposure exercises, however, would typically begin with an item on the SUDS rated at least a 3 or 4. Once treatment commences and the patient is familiar with the procedures, you could then assign the patient to complete additional exposure trials for all items falling at or below the level of the item faced in each session (i.e., if an item faced in session was rated a 4, the patient can then be assigned that item, as well as any additional items at 4 or below, for homework).

As treatment progresses, you and the patient can then collaboratively select a representative item from each level (e.g., SUDS ratings of 5, 6, 7) for the in-session exposure exercise, with any additional items at that level then being completed by the patient between/outside of the sessions. This process should be flexible however, so that (1) if the patient struggles with an item, it can be repeated in a future session, and (2) if the patient encounters an item (e.g., at a higher SUDS rating or unanticipated) that he is nevertheless willing to face, he is free to do so. This second point may be particularly relevant, as newer data (e.g., Kircanski et al., 2012) suggest that random and variable exposure may produce outcomes similar to traditional exposure. Moreover, greater emotion variability during exposure, which includes the ups and the downs of fear as opposed to pure habituation, may actually serve to enhance patient outcomes.

# HOMEWORK

## Review of the Rationale

Review once again the importance of practice in learning a new skill and the strong connection between homework compliance and treatment outcome. You can also remind the patient of the principle of collaborative empiricism and note that the data he collects and brings back to the sessions will play a major role in shaping the treatment—including which triggers will be targeted and how much time should be spent working on them—both within and between the sessions. If the patient has thus far been mainly compliant with completing, you can reinforce these efforts and encourage the patient to keep working hard, as efforts made now will help to build momentum, enhance treatment outcome, and help prevent relapse once the treatment has ended.

If the patient has not been compliant with the assignments thus far, you can remind him that it is normal to struggle with completing the homework. Be sure to review the problem-solving strategies that were covered during the homework check at the beginning of the session. In addition, you and the patient can collaborate to anticipate any potential challenges that could come up in the week ahead that might interfere with the patient's success in completing the assignment. Link the homework assignment to the patient's treatment goals, making sure that the patient sees the connection and therefore views the assignments as important, useful, and fairly easy to implement.

If the patient has enlisted the help of a coach, you can check to see how this arrangement has been working out, and once again, save a few minutes to check in with the coach as well (or obtain consent from the patient to check in with the coach between sessions). If necessary, remind the coach about how best to be of help to the patient (i.e., encourage and remind the patient of the treatment contract versus coerce and/or give reassurance) in order to maximize the benefits and minimize the costs of using a coach. If you will be acting as a coach to the patient between sessions (i.e., offering phone support between sessions), remind the patient about the rules of the phone supports (e.g., frequency, length, and format) and confirm when the next coaching session will begin.

## New Assignments

As has been the case in each of the previous treatment sessions, be sure to have the patient review the notes taken during this session and each of the previous sessions (especially if the patient did not demonstrate adequate understanding during the review at the beginning of the session), as well as reread any handouts previously assigned, and return with a summary and/or questions. You can also provide the patient with a printout (or photocopy) of the list of items that have been generated for the exposure hierarchy thus far and the SUDS. You can ask the patient to review both in order to determine if any adjustments are necessary before the hierarchy is finalized.

You should also ask the patient to continue to self-monitor the OCD symptoms, paying particular attention to any new triggers or patterns that may emerge between sessions. Depending on how well the patient completed the self-monitoring assignment between sessions, you should also remind him of any adjustments that should be made (e.g., when, where, and how the self-monitoring will be completed) and also ensure that he has enough copies of the Self-Monitoring Form (see Appendix B, Form 4). Finally, if a self-help book was assigned to augment the treatment, the patient can be asked to either start or continue reading it.

As was the case after assigning the homework at the end of the previous sessions, you should check to make sure that the patient agrees on the usefulness and importance of the assignments and sees their connection to the broader goals of treatment. If the patient does not agree that this would be a useful assignment, cannot see the connection of the assignment to the broader treatment goal(s), or struggled to complete the homework last time, you can address these issues before moving ahead. You can also normalize the fact that it can take some time to get the hang of it all and emphasize that making a strong and consistent *effort* is what is most important at this stage.

## RAPPORT AND ALLIANCE BUILDING: FEEDBACK, SUMMARY, AND TAKE-HOME MESSAGE

By now you and the patient should be accustomed to the notion of finishing the session with a discussion of feedback on the treatment thus far, as well as anything that could be changed to improve it. In this case, it can be particularly helpful to elicit feedback from the patient on the concept of SUDS, the items generated for the exposure hierarchy, and the road ahead in therapy. This promotes an atmosphere of collaboration and in so doing, not only helps to maintain rapport, trust, and a strong working alliance, but also explicitly encourages the patient to share in the responsibility for the treatment outcome. You should also be prepared to give feedback to the patient, starting with any positives observed, while also including constructive feedback on things that the patient can correct.

You and the patient can then take turns (with the patient starting) at summarizing the main points of the session, so that you can check the patient's understanding of the materials presented and see if the patient understood the main points. If the patient's summary is incomplete or inaccurate, you can add additional thoughts and/or make corrections to the summary, while being sure to check in with the patient to get agreement. Once you and the patient agree on the summary, you should wrap up by once again asking her for the take-home message from the session (e.g., "Based on what we covered in our session today, what have you learned and how will this change how you live your life?"). Asking this question reinforces the notion that the material covered in each session is not only important but can also have a practical impact on the patient's life. It can also be logically connected to the homework assignment given for the week in order to help facilitate transporting the material to outside of the office.

---

## TAKE-HOME MESSAGE FROM TREATMENT SESSION 3

Treatment Session 3 serves as a bridge between the foundational sessions (treatment Sessions 1 and 2) and the start of Ex/RP. In so doing, it provides time for a review of the CBT model of OCD and the rationale for Ex/RP.

By reviewing this material, you can ensure that the patient understands what has led to the maintenance of his symptoms, what he needs to do in order to feel better, and why he needs to do it. Although reviewing the materials covered may take a little more time, it allows for misconceptions and misunderstandings to be clarified and for any motivational issues or resistances to the treatment (or treatment model) to be addressed. Thus, by building a strong foundation up front, you have a place to return to for the remainder of the course of treatment, particularly when any "roadblocks" are encountered, as these are often due to a misunderstanding of the theory, model, or rationale. In addition, many patients feel empowered, motivated, and hopeful once they understand the theory, model, and rationale for treatment.

This session also provides you with an opportunity to transition the therapeutic relationship from information gathering from the patient to a more active collaboration in treatment planning with the patient. In particular, this transition occurs by customizing the treatment plan to address the patient's specific symptoms, via (1) creating a SUDS with anchors unique to the patient's life experience, and then (2) applying this scale to a list of the patient's unique situations, triggers, and obsessive thoughts in order to create the exposure hierarchy that will serve as the backbone for the remainder of the treatment.

# CHAPTER 10

# Treatment Session 4

## SESSION COMPONENTS

- Check on symptoms
  - Optional: Provide and score self-report measure(s)
- Review of the homework
  - Self-monitoring
  - Notes from the previous session (optional)
  - Psychoeducational handouts (optional)
    - CBT model of OCD
    - NIH Fact Sheet on Obsessive–Compulsive Disorder
  - Self-help book assignment (optional)
- Quick review of the CBT model of OCD, the rationale for CBT for OCD, and the concept of SUDS
- Review and finalize the exposure hierarchy
- Motivational enhancement
- Prepare for Ex/RP
- Provide a rough outline of how future sessions will be structured
- Introduce the notion of ritual prevention between sessions
- Homework
  - Review of the rationale
  - New assignments
- Rapport and alliance building: Feedback, summary, and a take-home message

## MATERIALS NEEDED

- Self-report measure(s)
- Dry-erase board, easel, or clip board for you to use
- Clip board for the patient to take notes during the session
- Copy of master list of hierarchy items with SUDS ratings

- Handouts/forms for homework
  - Self-Monitoring Forms
  - Copy of finalized hierarchy items with SUDS ratings
  - Decisional Balance Form
  - Self-help book recommendations (optional)

## CHECK ON SYMPTOMS

At this point, the patient can expect to be asked for a report on the severity of her OCD symptoms, the amount of effort she has been being put into the treatment, and the level of success she has had in managing her OCD symptoms since the last session. As in previous sessions, ideally, these scores will be immediately entered into a chart and then a spreadsheet program, where they can be graphed and then reviewed with the patient, so that she can receive immediate feedback on how the treatment is progressing. You and the patient can examine the ratings together and note any connections between the amount of effort put into the treatment, the level of success and control over the symptoms, and the overall OCD symptom severity. You can then reinforce the patient for any improvements observed or normalize any plateaus or slips in the treatment progress and reframe them (e.g., as tests of the patient's skills and resolve and as reminders of the need to continue to work hard every day in order to change the course of the disorder), and problem-solve as necessary (e.g., assess level of motivation and insight, homework compliance, comorbidity issues, psychosocial stressor changes).

## OPTIONAL: PROVIDE AND SCORE SELF–REPORT MEASURE(S)

If the patient has been completing a brief, empirically based, self-report measure of OCD (e.g., the OCI-R; see Appendix C, Form 11) at the start of certain sessions (e.g., weekly, monthly) and is due to complete one at this session, it is advisable to have him complete it just prior to the start of the session. It can then be scored at the start of the session, and feedback can be provided to him. If the score has decreased, it will allow the patient to see objectively that the treatment is progressing. This can enhance motivation and treatment compliance. If the score has not changed (or increased), it will allow you and the patient to have a discussion (i.e., problem-solve) about how to get the treatment back on track. In addition, specific items from the self-report can be used as a launching point for a discussion of particularly challenging situations/triggers that may be used for future exposure exercises.

## REVIEW OF THE HOMEWORK

### Self-Monitoring

If the patient completed the self-monitoring assignment, be sure to continue to reinforce his efforts by offering praise and reviewing any new symptoms that were not previously discussed. You can also provide corrective feedback on how to improve the monitoring, if necessary. Finally, be sure to ask about what may have been *left off* of the form (i.e., if any rituals were not recorded this week or if any rituals were prevented). If rituals have been left off, you can remind the patient that *all* rituals should be recorded and problem-solve if necessary. If rituals have been prevented, you can reinforce this effort (e.g., praise the patient for his hard work).

## Notes from the Previous Session (Optional)

If the patient took notes during the previous session and was asked to review the notes between sessions for homework, you can check whether she completed this task and if so, review any questions or comments she had about them. If the patient failed to complete the assignment, you can review the rationale for the assignment, assess what got in the way, collaborate with her to determine whether the assignment is worth repeating, and if so, problem-solve to ensure that the assignment will be completed before the next session.

## Psychoeducational Handouts (Optional)

If the patient was asked to review any psychoeducational handouts (e.g., the CBT model of OCD, the NIH OCD Fact Sheet) for homework, be sure to check whether she completed these tasks. If so, you can ask her for a summary of the main points and answer any questions or comments she had about them. If the patient failed to complete the assignment, you can review the rationale for the assignment, assess what got in the way, collaborate with her to determine whether the assignment is worth repeating, and if so, problem-solve to ensure that the assignment will be completed before the next session.

## Self–Help Book Assignment (Optional)

If the patient was assigned a self-help book and has already started reading it, you can ask him for a summary of the main points and ask whether he has any questions based on what he has read thus far. If the patient failed to complete the assignment, you can review the rationale for using a self-help book to augment the therapy, assess what got in the way, collaborate with him to determine whether the assignment is worth repeating, and if so, problem-solve to ensure that the assignment will be completed before the next session

# QUICK REVIEW OF THE CBT MODEL OF OCD, RATIONALE FOR CBT FOR OCD, AND THE CONCEPT OF SUDS

Ask if the patient has any questions about the CBT model of OCD and if so, answer them. You can then ask the patient to give a brief summary of the CBT model of OCD. By now, he should be able to explain the model with relatively little effort. If the patient is able to summarize the model with minimal or no corrections, you can then ask him to explain the rationale for CBT for OCD. You should ensure that this discussion is tied to the goals of treatment, which include (1) having patients gradually, systematically, and repeatedly face the various situations, triggers, and thoughts they have been avoiding, (2) without doing the things they have typically done to mitigate their thoughts or feelings of anxiety, so that (3) they develop a new relationship with her thoughts and, in so doing, (4) learn new things about the nature of their anxiety—all of which ultimately

(5) helps to weaken the link between the various situations, triggers, and thoughts and their feelings of anxiety. If the patient is able to explain the rationale with minimal or no corrections needed, you can then ask him to explain the concept of SUDS and how it fits with the rationale for CBT for OCD. Aim to be Socratic rather than didactic during these reviews, thereby making the discussion as interactive as possible.

If the patient demonstrates a clear grasp of all of these concepts, you can reinforce her efforts and move on to the finalization of the final exposure hierarchy. If the patient does not appear to understand the model, the rationale for treatment, or the concept of SUDS, you can briefly review them again and also reassign a review of the handouts and session notes for homework. It is very important that patients have a solid understanding of the model, rationale, and concept of SUDS before treatment begins, as doing so helps patients (1) become more objective observers of their symptoms, (2) identify and correct maladaptive behaviors (e.g., avoidance and rituals) during the treatment, and (3) stay motivated to continue with treatment during the more challenging times (e.g., lapses, particularly difficult exposure assignments, relapse prevention).

## REVIEW AND FINALIZE THE EXPOSURE HIERARCHY

If the patient's hierarchy items and SUDS ratings were entered into an electronic database, you should have the file open and ready for any fine-tuning based on the patient's review of the items between sessions. Often patients will adjust one or more of the SUDS ratings for specific items after seeing all of the items arranged in the hierarchy. In addition, patients often report that an item or two was omitted during the generation of the hierarchy items in the previous session. Therefore, you can ask if the patient thought of any additional items to be added to the hierarchy. If so, these items can be given a SUDS rating and then added to the hierarchy, which can then be resorted into descending order. If not, you can ask if the patient reviewed the copy of the master list of hierarchy items generated during the previous session, as well as the SUDS scale and anchors. Either way, you should then ask if she would like to make any adjustments in the rankings before considering the hierarchy to be final. If any adjustments need to be made, you can make them immediately and then print a copy of the new version for her.

If no adjustments need to be made, you can present the patient with a clean and sorted copy of the hierarchy created during the last session. You should make sure that the column with the ratings is dated, as the hierarchy items will be re-rated in future sessions (with the new ratings placed in new columns), to assess where progress is being made and where problems need to be addressed (see Figure 10.1 for an example, and see Appendix B, Form 9, for a blank Hierarchy Construction Worksheet). Finally, be sure to get the patient to "officially approve" the final hierarchy (in terms of content and SUDS ratings) before commencing with Ex/RP, as the hierarchy will serve as the backbone for the rest of the treatment.

## MOTIVATIONAL ENHANCEMENT

At this point in the treatment, many patients experience mixed emotions (i.e., ambivalence) about engaging in Ex/RP. On the one hand, they often can see the destruction and disability that their

| Item | SUDS (Date: 1/1/16) | SUDS (Date: ) | SUDS (Date: ) | SUDS (Date: ) |
|---|---|---|---|---|
| Using public toilet | 100 | | | |
| Touching floor (busy area) | 99 | | | |
| Touching bathroom door handle (inside) | 95 | | | |
| Touching bathroom faucet handles | 90 | | | |
| Touching urinal handle | 85 | | | |
| Touching inside of garbage can | 80 | | | |
| Lying down on office floor | 75 | | | |
| Touching seat cushion on public chair | 70 | | | |
| Handling money | 70 | | | |
| Touching bathroom door handle (outer) | 65 | | | |
| Touching office door knob | 60 | | | |
| Using public telephone | 55 | | | |
| Touching outside of garbage can | 50 | | | |
| Touching keyboard | 50 | | | |
| Touching seatback on public chair | 45 | | | |
| Touching elevator buttons | 45 | | | |
| Touching light switch | 40 | | | |
| Touching floor (corner of room) | 30 | | | |

**FIGURE 10.1.** Sample Hierarchy Construction Worksheet from treatment Session 4.

disorder is causing in their lives, are eager to rid themselves of the OCD, and understand that exposure will help them to accomplish this goal. On the other hand, they are often highly anxious about having to confront their most feared triggers, situations, and thoughts—all while giving up their most comforting rituals. As such, interventions that increase motivation can prepare patients adequately for the cognitive, behavioral, and emotional challenges that lie ahead and in so doing, improve treatment retention, engagement, and outcome.

For example, in today's wired and reality-based television show world, many patients may have already read about exposure or seen television shows or videos in which exposure therapy is carried out. Unfortunately, not all of the content of the web is accurate, and many television shows will air only the most dramatic clips from hours of treatment with the most extreme cases. Therefore, patients might also have some misgivings or misunderstandings about how Ex/RP works and what they can expect. Also, some patients may report that they have already tried Ex/RP—either on their own or with the aid of another therapist in the past. Unfortunately, this can, at times, be more problematic than preparing a patient for treatment who has never tried Ex/RP before because it must now be determined what part of the previous course of therapy was not helpful.

As such, interventions that aim to increase motivation should target preconceived notions and expectations about therapy, address past failed attempts, and attack ambivalence directly. In so doing, treatment retention, engagement, and ultimately outcome may be improved. For example, with regard to preconceived notions, providing the patient with psychoeducation is often helpful. Patients can be asked Socratically about the objectivity and accuracy of television programs and information on the Internet in order to highlight potential problems in relying solely on these types of media as a basis for drawing conclusions about the treatment. With regard to previous treatments, you will need to determine how much of a role the previous therapist may have played in the outcome (e.g., examining how the procedures were carried out, correcting any misinformation given) and how much of a role the patient may have played in the outcome (e.g., understanding of the rationale, motivation at the time, engagement in homework, the presence of other confounding factors). In these cases, it may also prove beneficial to have the patient sign a release of information form so that the former therapist may be contacted to obtain ideas about the treatment that the patient omitted.

Finally, as mentioned in Chapter 7, one of the most common methods used to target ambivalence directly to enhance motivation for change is by completing a Decisional Balance Worksheet with the patient (see Figure 10.2 and Figure 7.2 in Chapter 7 for examples; a blank copy of the worksheet is available in Appendix B, Form 2). Recall that this is done by eliciting from the patient the perceived costs and benefits of making a change (e.g., engaging in exposure therapy) versus maintaining the status quo (e.g., continuing to avoid and engage in rituals). The patient can be encouraged to consider past, current, and future costs and benefits, in all domains (e.g., medical, social, occupational, psychological). Ideally, by acknowledging and addressing all of the short-term costs of engaging exposure and ritual prevention (e.g., a temporary increase in anxiety and urge to ritualize) that make it unappealing, as well as expanding on all of the long-term benefits (e.g., a life without having to do rituals, increased mood and esteem, more time to pursue valued activities) that can be reaped if the patient is willing to try it, the patient's ambivalence will diminish. It's important to remember, however, that a patient's motivation can also fluctuate *throughout the course of treatment*. As a result, it is a good idea to revisit the patient's motivation level again now (i.e., review the Decisional Balance Worksheet or complete a new one, if necessary), and you may also have to revisit motivational-enhancing strategies regularly throughout the treatment in order to keep it progressing.

## PREPARE FOR EX/RP

Prior to commencing with Ex/RP, it is important that you make clear how the exposure sessions will be structured and what will be expected of the patient—both within and between the sessions. Taking the time to inform the patient about what to expect—and what is expected of

| | Benefits/Pros (short term and long term) | Costs/Cons (short-term and long-term) |
|---|---|---|
| **Do not make a change** (e.g., "Do not give Ex/RP a try and continue to manage my OCD the same way I always have.") | • *Won't be setting myself up for disappointment if it does not work* <br> • *Won't have to confront my problems* <br> • *Less effort required* | • *Symptoms likely won't change (and have been getting worse)* <br> • *Financial problems because I can't work* <br> • *No partner because I can't date* <br> • *Disapproval from my friends and family* <br> • *Putting my health at risk* |
| **Make a change** (e.g., "Give Ex/RP a try so I can learn to manage my OCD in new way.") | • *Will give myself a chance at a better life* <br> • *Will learn skills to manage my symptoms* <br> • *Will improve relationships with family and friends* <br> • *Will have decreased job problems* <br> • *Will feel less anxious and depressed in the future (if it works!)* | • *Will have to invest time into the treatment (e.g., attend sessions and do homework)* <br> • *Will feel more stressed and anxious (in the short term?!)* |

**FIGURE 10.2.** Sample Decisional Balance Worksheet.

her—allows for a framework to be created for the remainder of the treatment while also clarifying any misconceptions she may have about how Ex/RP works. In addition, the patient will be able to understand how each session is designed to help her overcome a different aspect of her OCD and, if she works hard, can lead to a time when she will no longer need treatment (i.e., by facing and mastering the item at the top of their hierarchy). This can help motivate patients and instill hope by showing them that the end is in sight.

Referring to the copy of the finalized hierarchy that you provided to the patient, you can inform her that the in-session Ex/RP phase of treatment will begin at the next session. Next, you and the patient can together review the items on her finalized hierarchy and select a representative item for each major SUDS level in the hierarchy to be conducted in session (e.g., if there are three items rated 4/10, in most cases you and the patient should only select one of these for the in-session Ex/RP). The expectation is that as the patient successfully faces an item of a certain SUDS value in session, she should then be able to repeat that item, along with items of the same value, on her own outside of the session. If this turns out to not be the case, then the other item(s) of equal SUDS value can be used for in-session Ex/RP in future sessions.

You and the patient can then select the item to be used for the initial Ex/RP session. Some patients might feel particularly motivated and wish to start with the highest item on their hierarchy. Although this may seem like a good idea, it is often wise to hold off on this urge and select an item with a lower SUDS rating for the very first Ex/RP session, especially for patients who have never tried Ex/RP before. By "stacking the deck" to increase the odds of a successful first exposure, you can help increase the patient's motivation to engage in the treatment, as well as the patient's confidence in the notion that the treatment will help them. In addition, a failed initial exposure may cause a rupture in the therapeutic alliance, a loss of credibility in the treatment, and a decrease in motivation to continue.

Conversely, other patients may feel particularly anxious and therefore may wish to start with the absolute lowest item on their hierarchy (e.g., an item rated 1/10 or 2/10). Although this may also seem to be a good idea, it is often prudent to hold off on this urge in all but the most severe cases. Items with very low SUDS ratings may fail to activate the patient's fear structure or be potent enough to generate enough anxiety to demonstrate the concept of habituation. As a result, patients may fail to integrate any new, corrective information into their fear structure or experience the feeling of relief from their anxiety without engaging in rituals, each of which is highly important when establishing a template for future exposure sessions. On rare occasions, however (e.g., if the patient has expressed ambivalence about Ex/RP or has had setbacks in the past), starting with a lower item can be considered, if it can be used to build the patient's confidence and motivation and create some momentum in the treatment.

In most instances, however, patients often will agree to face lower-level items on their own, once they have an idea of how Ex/RP works. As a result, you can suggest to the patient that the best place to start is with an item that is from the lower-middle section of the hierarchy (e.g., approximate SUDS value of 4 or 5 out of 10). By selecting an item from within this SUDS range, the patient should benefit in a number of ways. First, he may feel relief that he will not have to face his worst fears right away. Second, he may perceive these items as having less "severe" consequences than items with a higher SUDS rating, which may enhance his willingness to engage in the treatment. Third, using an item of moderate SUDS for exposure should be anxiety-provoking enough to activate the patient's fear structure (i.e., allow the patient to access his feared thoughts/consequences and experience the urge to engage in rituals), yet manageable enough to allow him to successfully resist the urge to ritualize while at the same time experiencing his feelings of anxiety diminish (via habituation). This will allow the patient to learn something new during the session about his fears (i.e., corrects negative predictions) as well as the need to ritualize (i.e., don't have to do rituals to feel less anxious)—while being at a level that will not be overly stressful (i.e., he will be able to recompose himself and go on with his day after the session and as a result, feel good about the outcome). As a result, the patient will leave the first exposure session with a sense of mastery over the task and increased confidence in his ability to successfully face items of higher SUDS ratings in future sessions.

As mentioned above, if there are several items all in the same SUDS ratings range (e.g., 4–5/10), only one should be selected for the first exposure. When deciding which item to select, however, you should maintain a collaborative stance with the patient and ask if there is an item from the group that she would like to select for the first exposure. In so doing, the patient should feel more involved—and therefore invested—in the treatment process.

Many patients will begin to feel anxious after selecting the starting item for Ex/RP, as this serves as a reminder that they will soon have to start confronting their fears without using the tools they have relied on for so long to feel better. As such, you will want to normalize this response and link it to the CBT model covered earlier in the treatment (e.g., patients can expect their anxiety to rise as avoidance is blocked and triggers are gradually confronted, with longer periods of avoidance generating higher levels of anticipatory anxiety). You may also want to engage the patient in a discussion of how patients who experience an increased level of anticipatory anxiety commonly also experience a temporary rise in the OCD symptoms. This can lead to urges to avoid the start of the in-session exposure, such as by coming in with other "urgent" topics to discuss, arriving late for sessions, or avoiding treatment altogether (e.g., canceling appointments). In addition, you can instruct the patient to not take any special advance "precautions" (i.e., engage in "preventative" rituals before the Ex/RP session) to counter the feared consequences of the upcoming exposure task (e.g., saying a special prayer before the session, seeking reassurance, wearing special clothes).

## PROVIDE A ROUGH OUTLINE OF HOW FUTURE SESSIONS WILL BE STRUCTURED

Explain to the patient that the focus of the next 10 sessions will be on facing items from her hierarchy, one at a time, starting with the item that was just selected (see the previous section). Inform the patient that, as a collaborator, she will always have a say in each exposure and will never be forced to do anything against her will. Also, inform the patient that, starting with the next session, the standard agenda will involve having a brief check-in, followed immediately by Ex/RP as early as possible in the session, to allow adequate time for habituation and processing of the exposure (i.e., new learning) to occur.

Acknowledge that exposure is like "a bitter pill": it does not "taste" good going down (i.e., it feels uncomfortable at first) but ultimately will help her to feel better. As a result, in the short term, the patient should be prepared to feel worse (i.e., more anxious) before feeling better (i.e., less anxious). You can add, however, that if the patient follows the rules of treatment, the exposures should get easier with each practice. In addition, you can remind the patient that you will be there as a role model and a coach both in the sessions and between the sessions, helping the patient to stay focused, demonstrating how to do the exposure exercises (if necessary, at the start of treatment), and problem-solving any difficulties she faces when trying exposure exercises on her own.

Inform the patient that each item faced during the office visit will then be assigned for homework between the sessions. Explain that the between-session Ex/RP practices should be treated in the exact same way as an office visit (e.g., structured, deliberate, and long enough for habituation and/or new learning to occur). Remind the patient of the role that completing the between-session Ex/RP assignments has in treatment outcome and suggest that the patient practice Ex/RP at least once each day for as long as it takes to habituate and learn something new about the trigger, obsessive thoughts, appraisals, or rituals. As mentioned previously, it is often useful to use a metaphor or analogy here (e.g., learning to manage OCD symptoms is like learning a new language: it takes regular practice to become "fluent") in order to emphasize that the outcome of the treatment largely depends on the amount of work the patient does between sessions.

Remind the patient of the CBT principle of collaborative empiricism and encourage him to view the between-session homework assignments as an opportunity to "field test" the Ex/RP exercise that was completed during the session, in order to "gather data" on how well the results achieved during the session generalize into the "real world" outside of your office. As a result, rather than being an "assignment" that the patient completes for *you*, the "homework" in Ex/RP involves having the patient collect data for *himself*—by recording the results of any between-session Ex/RP practices on an Ex/RP Practice Record (see Figure 10.3; a blank version of the Ex/RP Practice Record is available in Appendix B, Form 10)—which can then be brought into the next therapy session for review and discussion *with* the therapist, if necessary.

Patients will often ask whether they should do additional exposures to other items (e.g., those

---

**Name:** Joe Smith                                                     **Date:** June 1, 2015

Exposure item/situation/imaginal scenario: Touching outside of my garbage can (at home).

Exposure start time: 6:30 PM          Exposure end time: 7:15 PM

Pre-SUDS (Anticipatory Anxiety): 70          Predicted Max. SUDS: 90

Feared outcome and/or consequences (be specific!): I will get sick (stomach virus) by the end of the evening and spread this to my wife and children, who will also get sick, causing us all to miss school/work! I won't be able to handle my anxiety about this. I will lose control!

Strength of belief in feared outcome before starting (0–10): 6

SUDS at start: 80   SUDS at 10 minutes: 65   SUDS at 20 minutes: 55   SUDS at 30 minutes: 45

SUDS at 40 minutes: 20   SUDS after 50 minutes: N/A   SUDS at end: 20   Max. SUDS: N/A

Results of feared outcome: To be determined!          Belief in feared outcome at end (0–10): 3

Alternative beliefs about the feared outcome and/or consequences: Touching the can, while unpleasant, ill not make me sick, and it's very unlikely that I can spread the germs to endanger my family members. I may feel anxious, but I can handle it.

Strength of belief in alternative beliefs (0–10): 7

Urge to ritualize at end (0–10): 4          Willingness to engage in ritual prevention (0–10): 10

Comments about this practice, including anything new that was learned and any difficulties that were encountered: This was the toughest exposure yet! I never thought I'd be able to touch that garbage can again—especially without washing afterward. But I was ready for the challenge and feel great (now that it's over!). I am learning that my thoughts are only powerful when I am nervous!

---

**FIGURE 10.3.** Sample Ex/RP Practice Record.

lower or higher than the item assigned) for homework. In general, you can encourage the patient to engage in as many exposure exercises as he wants, as long as they are well planned (e.g., structured so that something new can be learned and long enough for habituation to occur). However, you should be cautious about encouraging exposure to items of *higher* SUDS ratings than the item assigned, especially before the patient's anxiety has been extinguished to the current item being worked on in treatment (i.e., the item only generates minimal anxiety, such as a SUDS rating of 2 or less), for at least two Ex/RP trials in a row.

It should be noted once again, however, that emerging data (e.g., Kircanski et al., 2012; Culver, Stoyanova, & Craske, 2012) is beginning to challenge whether the traditional exposure paradigm is necessary to achieve clinical improvement. Given that this data is relatively new and limited at this time, however, you should only consider allowing the patient to face items of a higher SUDS value on his own between sessions after a few sessions. This is especially the case if they present themselves "naturalistically" in the patient's life—once the patient has demonstrated that he has a solid grasp of the rationale and mechanics of exposure. Though more challenging, this will allow the patient to practice dealing with potential triggers in a manner that more closely matches the "real world" and thus should allow treatment gains to generalize and build skills that may aid in relapse prevention.

Explain to the patient that in each treatment session following the next one, the two of you will either repeat an item (if still causing anxiety) or move up a level on the patient's hierarchy. As was the case for selecting the first item for exposure, if there is a cluster of items with the same SUDS rating on the next level up, the next item will be selected in a collaborative manner. As mentioned earlier, you and the patient may even want to make a rough plan as to which items will be used for the in-session Ex/RP exercises in each session, for the entire 10 sessions. The goal, however, should be to get to the most challenging item(s) as quickly as possible, so that the greater proportion of the Ex/RP sessions can be dedicated to facing the patient's most challenging triggers together and problem-solving any roadblocks.

Many patients find it difficult to imagine that they will be able to face their most anxiety-provoking item within five or six sessions (i.e., if starting with an item rated 4 or 5 out of 10 on the SUDS, ideally within the next five or six sessions, the treatment will target an item rated at a 10). Suggest that the patient avoid making any negative predictions and keep an open mind about how the treatment will progress. At the same time, emphasize that each patient's treatment progresses at a different pace, and, as such, the plan will not be written in stone (i.e., items may be repeated, added, or modified in some way, based on how the treatment is progressing). In addition, you can stress the importance of staying in the moment and working on the current task at hand, rather than worrying about the challenges that lie ahead (i.e., fixating on how difficult it will be to face the items on the top of the hierarchy before even commencing with the exposure practices).

Be sure to allow enough time to answer any questions that the patient has about Ex/RP or the structure of the next 10 sessions (including between-session assignments). Once all questions and concerns have been addressed, you can ask the patient to "contract" (verbally, but if necessary, in writing) to the treatment (i.e., agree to rules, expectations, and roles) before proceeding. Finally, you should determine whether any special materials (i.e., trigger items) are needed for the exposure exercise that will be conducted at the next session and, if so, collaborate with the patient to determine which of you will be responsible for obtaining them. Many therapists who treat OCD using Ex/RP end up building an "exposure kit" over time that contains items commonly found on the patient's hierarchies. At other times, an item will be specific to a particular patient's OCD, which the patient will have to bring in (e.g., a photo of a loved one).

If the patient has enlisted the help of a coach, you can bring the coach in at this point to (1) check on how the coaching role has been working out; (2) ask about any changes noted in the patient's OCD symptoms; (3) inform the coach of the start of Ex/RP next session, along with what to expect and how best to help (encourage and remind the patient of the treatment contract vs. coerce and/or give reassurance) in order to maximize the benefits and minimize the costs of using one; and (4) introduce the notion of ritual prevention, starting after this session (see the next section).

## INTRODUCE THE NOTION OF RITUAL PREVENTION BETWEEN SESSIONS

Before concluding this session, you should alert the patient to the importance of striving for 100% ritual prevention between sessions. This can be done by first reminding the patient of the CBT model of OCD and then presenting her with a rationale and instructions for ritual prevention, using specific examples for the patient's particular symptoms. You should also allow time to address any questions or concerns about this from the patient or the coach.

Begin by discussing the important role of rituals in maintaining the patient's OCD (e.g., prevent disconfirmation of fears, generate short-term relief from anxiety, increase importance of triggers). Then remind the patient of how engaging in these rituals has not only failed to eliminate the OCD symptoms, but instead has contributed to the worsening of the rituals, as they typically become more frequent and elaborate over time, all while providing less and less relief. Emphasize how critical it therefore becomes for the patient to begin striving to eliminate any and all rituals— starting right after the current session.

Explain that while initially anxiety-provoking, ritual prevention will provide several benefits in the long term, including (1) discovering that the ability to prevent rituals is not dichotomous (i.e., either one can or cannot do it), but rather success at ritual prevention is dimensional (i.e., patients have times when they are better at it and times when they struggle more at it), and the factors that make it more challenging can be addressed to improve her results; (2) maximizing the upcoming exposure exercises by eliminating an overall sense of reassurance (e.g., "I can do these exposures because I'll be able to ritualize at home"); and (3) creating opportunities for new learning to occur (e.g., "I will eventually need to ritualize in order to feel better").

Some patients will point out that engaging in ritual prevention is easier said than done; if it were as simple as just telling themselves to stop ritualizing, they would not need to be in treatment. You can validate this concern, while at the same time inquiring into how much of a consistent effort the patient has put into trying to do just that. In addition, you can note that the patient is now being encouraged to do this as one step within a larger treatment plan, after having now learned about the CBT model of OCD and how symptoms are perpetuated. Finally, you can note that the patient is only being asked to commit to *strive* for 100% ritual prevention, and add that it is understood that the patient is likely to "slip up" in his efforts, especially at the start. You and the patient can even anticipate these slips and problem-solve in advance by having the patient agree to (1) view any slips as challenges, (2) record any slips on the self-monitoring form, (3) ask for help from you or their coach (if they have one), and (4) make a plan on how to resist any urges to ritualize and (5) what to do in the event of a slip (e.g., immediately record the incident on the monitoring form and/or proceed to "undo" the slip by re-exposing themselves immediately to the situation or thought that generated the rituals).

Some patients may also point out that what they are being asked to do is much more extreme/excessive than what "normal" people do in their daily lives. You should acknowledge this complaint, while also noting how, given the severity of the patient's symptoms, another purpose of 100% ritual prevention is to "swing the patient's pendulum of tolerance/ability" during treatment to a level that is likely higher than that of people without OCD. The patient should understand that these rules will be loosened toward the end of treatment, and thus, the pendulum will likely swing back slightly and ultimately end up within the "normal" range.

Be certain to include specific examples that match the patient's particular symptom presentation. Although therapists differ on how "extreme" to make ritual prevention, in general you should start at the strictest level the patient is willing to tolerate—or is working toward as strict a level as possible, as quickly as possible, as the treatment progresses. For example, with respect to washing rituals, you might ask the patient to agree to temporarily "ban" washing with soap (and even rinsing with water) while he is in the active (exposure) phase of treatment. This ban could potentially cover everything from showering to hand washing to tooth brushing, and it might also include a ban on the use of hand sanitizers.

Needless to say, it is important for you to collaborate with the patient on these agreements. Compromises and exceptions should be made, especially (1) initially, to gain the patient's compliance with treatment and (2) at any time when medically indicated. As an example, some therapists will permit "supervised" showers (e.g., timed by the patient's coach, but not necessarily involving direct observation—see the next paragraph), as long as they are kept to a strict schedule and time limit (e.g., no more than 10 minutes, every one, two, or three days) and any showering rituals are prevented (e.g., specific washing routines, repeated washing of specific body parts). Other therapists will permit the limited use of certain toiletry or other hygiene products. Regardless of the strictness of the level of ritual prevention ultimately decided upon, you can remind the patient that what's most important is to be aware of the *function* of the activity he is about to engage in. In other words, the patient can begin to ask himself whether what he is about to do is aimed at reducing feelings of contamination and, if so, the patient should consider whether engaging in this action will get him toward his goal.

As mentioned earlier, the patient's compliance with ritual prevention between sessions may be enhanced if he has elected to use a coach to augment the therapy. If this is the case, the coach can be provided with instructions on how to be most helpful with this portion of the treatment. For example, in general, the coach should be available to the patient (especially initially) during any "high-risk" times (e.g., before eating, upon returning home, when coming into contact with loved ones), and specifically, at any time in which the patient experiences strong urges to ritualize that she feels unable to control on her own. Ideally, the coach will be available in person during these times, so that the patient can receive assistance in ritual prevention until the urge decreases to a more manageable level. Although it may seem obvious, it is important for you to emphasize that the coach should only attempt to aid in ritual prevention using encouragement and reminding the patient of the rationale and rules, and should never provide reassurance, argue with the patient, insult the patient, make threats, or attempt to physically restrain the patient. This is also a good time to again check to see how the coaching has been working out, and if necessary, help the coach and patient to problem-solve any issues. If you will be acting as a coach to the patient between sessions (i.e., offering phone support between sessions), remind the patient about the rules of the phone supports (e.g., frequency, length, and format) and confirm when the next coaching session will occur.

# HOMEWORK

## Review of the Rationale

Review once again the importance of practice in learning a new skill and the strong connection between homework compliance and positive treatment outcomes. You can also remind the patient of the principle of collaborative empiricism and note that the data he collects and brings back to the sessions will play a major role in shaping the treatment. If the patient has thus far mainly been compliant with completing the homework assignments, you can reinforce these efforts and encourage the patient to keep working hard. You should emphasize that, while challenging, the efforts made over the next phase of treatment will help to build momentum, enhance treatment outcome, and prevent relapse once the treatment has ended.

If the patient has not been compliant with completing the assignments thus far or seems hesitant about response prevention and/or the upcoming exposure sessions, you can remind him that it takes time and effort to do the treatment and that motivation and commitment can waiver over time. You can also state that it is normal to be anxious about giving up strategies that the patient believes have been useful (even when these strategies do not appear to be working) while facing the situations, objects, and thoughts that the patient has feared for so long. You should suggest that the patient review the treatment goal(s) for motivation and commit to putting in the maximum effort each day, knowing that the patient's actual success in this endeavor will vary from day to day—especially at the start of this phase. Be sure to emphasize the link between the homework assignment to the patient's broader treatment goals, making sure that the patient sees the connection and therefore views the assignments as important and useful, even if challenging to implement. If necessary, you can review what has gotten in the way thus far and make/adjust a plan to address these obstacles in the time before the next session. You and the patient can also try to anticipate any potential challenges that could arise in the week ahead that may interfere with the patient's success in completing the homework assignments.

## New Assignments

As has been the case in each of the previous sessions, you can have the patient review any notes taken during the session and in each of the previous sessions, and then return with a summary and/or questions. If the patient has continued to struggle to understand the model or rationale for treatment, you can consider having him review the handouts previously assigned one more time.

Ask the patient to continue to self-monitor the OCD symptoms, paying particular attention to any new triggers or patterns that may emerge between sessions. Depending on how well the patient has been completing the self-monitoring assignment between sessions, you can also remind her of any adjustments that should be made (e.g., when, where, and how the self-monitoring will be completed) and also ensure that she has enough copies of the Self-Monitoring Form (see Appendix B, Form 4). In addition, you can emphasize that from this point on the patient should be striving for 100% ritual prevention. In other words, the patient will continue to complete columns for triggers and/or obsessive thoughts and level of anxiety, but will strive to have as few entries as possible in the rituals column.

Be sure to provide the patient with a printout of the finalized hierarchy (or photocopy of the Hierarchy Construction Worksheet—see Appendix B, Form 9) and remind him that starting next session the two of you will begin to conduct in-session Ex/RP. In addition, if the first exposure trial requires an item unique to the patient (e.g., picture of a family member, contaminated object from home), you can remind the patient to bring this item in for the next session. Finally, if a self-help book was assigned to augment the treatment, the patient can be asked to continue reading it.

As was the case after assigning the homework at the end of the previous sessions, you can check to make sure that the patient agrees on the usefulness and importance of the assignments and sees their connection to the broader goals of treatment. If the patient does not agree that the homework will be useful, cannot see the importance that the assignment plays in achieving the broader treatment goal(s), or struggled to complete the homework last time, you should address these issues before moving ahead. Sometimes a review of the rationale or model will help. Other times a modification of the task with the patient's input may increase her willingness to try it. If the patient completed a Decisional Balance Worksheet (see Appendix B, Form 2) during this—or a previous—session, you can instruct her to review it if she is anxious about commencing Ex/RP. The bottom line, however, is that the patient's resistance should be discussed and addressed before moving ahead. Simply insisting that the patient complete the assignment will not likely be effective and would violate the collaborative nature of the treatment, whereas minimizing or ignoring lack of compliance will undermine the importance of the homework and may negatively impact treatment outcome.

## RAPPORT AND ALLIANCE BUILDING: FEEDBACK, SUMMARY, AND TAKE-HOME MESSAGE

As was the case for each of the previous sessions, be sure to continue to build rapport, trust, and a strong working alliance with the patient by eliciting feedback about what was liked and disliked about the session, your performance as a therapist, and how the therapy is progressing. In this way, patients will continue to experience the treatment as a collaborative process and hopefully share more in the responsibility for the treatment outcome. You can also give feedback to the patient about anything positive observed—either in this session or since the initial intake—while also providing constructive, corrective feedback if necessary. In this case, it can be helpful to elicit feedback from the patient on the final exposure hierarchy, the goal of striving for 100% ritual prevention, the upcoming first exposure session, and the road ahead in therapy.

Finally, you and the patient can then take turns (with the patient starting) at summarizing the main points of the session, so that you can check his understanding of the materials presented and see if he understood the main points. If the patient's summary is incomplete or inaccurate, you can add additional thoughts and/or make corrections to the summary, while being sure to check in with the patient in order to get agreement. Once you and the patient agree on the summary, you should wrap up by once again asking him for the take-home message from the session (e.g., "Based on what we covered in our session today, what have you learned and how will this change how you live your life?"). Asking this question reinforces the notion that the material covered in each session is not only important but can also have a practical impact on the patient's life. It should also be logically connected to the homework assignment given for the week to help facilitate transporting the material to outside of the office.

---

## TAKE-HOME MESSAGE FROM TREATMENT SESSION 4

Treatment Session 4 serves as both a consolidation and motivation-building session. In so doing, it provides time to ensure that the patient has a solid understanding of the CBT model of OCD, the rationale for CBT for OCD, and the concept of SUDS. It also encourages the patient to consider the role that he has played in maintaining his OCD symptoms, what he needs to do in order to get better, and how the final hierarchy will serve as the blueprint for the next 10 sessions in order to get the patient there. It then provides time to increase/maintain the patient's motivation to change by addressing any ambivalence that the patient has about making a change by exploring the costs and benefits in the short and long term of approaching things differently (i.e., engaging in Ex/RP). It then helps ameliorate any of the patient's anxiety about engaging in this change by finalizing the hierarchy as a team, providing an overview of how the Ex/RP sessions will be structured, collaborating on which item from the hierarchy to start with, and assigning an initial task of simply striving for 100% ritual prevention between sessions. Finally, you continue to build rapport and strengthen the treatment alliance by including the patient in all tasks in the session—from being interactive in the review of the material to making sure the patient approves the final hierarchy to soliciting feedback at the end of the session.

# CHAPTER 11

# Treatment Sessions 5–14

## *Ten Sessions of Exposure and Ritual Prevention*

This chapter outlines the foundation for the next 10 sessions of the treatment. For many patients, adhering to this foundation will be sufficient to help them achieve their treatment goals. In some cases, however, it will be important to augment or adjust this plan to suit the needs of a specific patient. For example, in some cases, you may decide to incorporate cognitive and/or metacognitive interventions into treatment, while in other cases, you may have to return to the use of motivational enhancement techniques to address decreases in the patient's motivation to engage in Ex/RP. Examples of these interventions are described in Chapter 14. In these instances, you can either add the desired intervention(s) to the core agenda for each session (outlined below) or delete one (or more) of these 10 sessions to substitute in a session (or more) with an entirely different agenda. What's most important is for you to be consistent in setting (and following!) an agenda that contains both general (e.g., agenda setting, homework assigning) and specific (e.g., Ex/RP, cognitive, and motivational techniques) evidence-based elements, while moving at a pace that matches each patient's specific abilities and needs.

## SESSION COMPONENTS

- Brief check on symptoms
  - Ratings of effort and success at 100% ritual prevention
  - Optional: Brief check on self-report measure(s)
- Brief review of the homework
  - Self-monitoring of OCD symptoms and whether successful at preventing rituals
  - Notes/handouts/questions from the previous session (optional)
  - Between-session *in vivo* and/or imaginal Ex/RP practices (Sessions 6–14)
  - Self-help book assignment (optional)
  - Item for Ex/RP (optional)
- Brief review of the CBT model of OCD and the rationale for exposure

- Brief check on the patient's motivation to engage in Ex/RP
  - Decisional Balance Worksheet (optional)
  - Create/review treatment contract (optional)
- Brief reminder of the session structure
- In-session Ex/RP: *In vivo* and/or imaginal
- Homework
  - Review of the rationale (Session 5 only)
  - New assignments
- Rapport and alliance building: Feedback, summary, and a take-home message
- Preparing for the home visit (optional at the end of Session 14 or at any point when deemed necessary)

## MATERIALS NEEDED

- Self-report measure(s)
- Dry-erase board, easel, or clip board for you to use
- Clip board for the patient to take notes during the session
- Copy of master list of hierarchy items with SUDS ratings
- Item(s) for in-session exposure
- Handouts/forms for homework
  - Self-Monitoring Forms
  - At-home Ex/RP Practice formsRecords
  - Self-help book recommendations (optional)

## BRIEF CHECK ON SYMPTOMS

Once the Ex/RP phase of treatment begins, you should make sure that the patient does not use the excessive asking of questions as a way to delay or avoid engaging in in-session exposure exercises.

In the interest of (1) maximizing the time available for in-session Ex/RP, (2) reinforcing any effort made between sessions to comply with homework assignments, and (3) transitioning the emphasis from between-session monitoring of symptoms to between-session active resisting/preventing of rituals, you should start by asking the patient to rate his effort and success at achieving 100% ritual prevention between sessions (using 0–10 scales), along with the now established self-report from the patient on his overall OCD severity. As in previous sessions, ideally, these scores will be immediately entered into a chart and then a spreadsheet program, where they can be graphed and reviewed with the patient, so that the patient can receive immediate feedback on how the treatment is progressing. From this session on, however, the emphasis would shift from the amount of effort put into the treatment and the level of success in managing the OCD symptoms to the amount of effort and success at achieving 100% ritual prevention. You and the patient should examine the ratings together and note any connections between the amount of effort put into ritual prevention, the level of success at ritual prevention, and the overall OCD severity. As in previous sessions, you should reinforce the patient for any improvements observed, or normalize any plateaus and/or slips in the treatment progress, reframe them (e.g., as tests of the patient's skills and resolve, and as reminders of the need to continue to work hard every day to change the course of the disorder), and then problem-solve as necessary (e.g., assess level of motivation and insight, homework compliance, comorbidity issues, psychosocial stressor changes).

### Optional: Brief Check on Self-Report Measure(s)

If the patient has been completing, a brief, empirically based, self-report measure of OCD (e.g., the OCI-R; see Appendix C, Form 11) at the start of certain sessions (e.g., weekly, monthly) and is due to complete one at this session, it is advisable to have the patient complete it just prior to the start of the session, so that it can be scored at the start of the session and feedback can be provided to the patient. As in previous sessions, treatment compliance and motivation can be enhanced if the patient can see objectively that progress is being made (i.e., the score has decreased). The measure may also be useful for generating a discussion on problem solving together if treatment progress has stalled (i.e., the score has not changed) or slipped (i.e., the score has increased). Specific items may also be used as a launching point for discussion of particularly challenging situations and triggers that may be used for future exposure exercises.

## BRIEF REVIEW OF THE HOMEWORK

As in the case with the brief check on symptoms (see above), you should be vigilant for patients who may use the asking of questions about the homework as a way to delay or avoid doing exposure exercises in session, in particular with exposure set to begin.

### Self-Monitoring of OCD Symptoms and Whether Successful at Preventing Rituals

Assuming that the patient has not been able to achieve 100% ritual prevention at this point, you can normalize this result, reinforce any efforts the patient made to complete the monitoring, and briefly review the entries completed by the patient on the Self-Monitoring Form (to see if any new triggers or symptoms emerged that were not previously mentioned). You can also ask if any rituals were not reported on the form and, if so, be sure to remind the patient that *all* rituals should be recorded and problem-solved if necessary. Finally, you can ask which (if any) rituals have been prevented, reinforce any progress made by the patient, and encourage the patient to continue monitoring all slips in the coming week.

### Notes/Handouts/Questions from the Previous Session (Optional)

If the patient took notes or was given any forms or handouts (e.g., the Decisional Balance Worksheet [see Appendix B, Form 2], a copy of the finalized hierarchy) to review between sessions, you can briefly check whether the patient completed these tasks and if so, ask the patient for a summary of the main points and/or answer any questions or comments the patient had about them. In addition, whenever you are using the Decisional Balance Worksheet as a homework assignment, be sure to pay particular attention to any additional costs and benefits the patient noted, so that a plan can be made for how the patient can address the costs and focus on the benefits when engaging in Ex/RP. Finally, if the patient took notes during the previous session and was asked to review the notes between sessions for homework, you can check whether the patient completed this task and if so, go over any questions or comments that arose while the patient was reviewing them. If the patient failed to complete the assignment, you can restore the rationale for the assignment, assess what got in the way, collaborate with the patient to determine whether the assignment is worth repeating, and if so, problem-solve to ensure that the assignment will be completed before the next session.

### Between-Session *In Vivo* and/or Imaginal Ex/RP Practices (Sessions 6–14)

Starting at the end of Session 5, be sure to give the patient several copies of the Ex/RP Practice Record (see Appendix B, Form 10) and review how to complete it, using the exposure exercise completed in each session as an example. Instruct the patient to practice Ex/RP each day between sessions, with the exercises targeting the item(s) completed in session, along with any other items from the hierarchy rated at the same SUDS level or below the item from the current session.

You and the patient (and coach, if applicable) should collaborate and agree on which items from the hierarchy the patient will work on for homework. It is advisable that you write these items on the Ex/RP Practice Record (see Appendix B, Form 10) as they are agreed upon, thereby avoiding any confusion. Encourage the patient to practice as much as possible each day, with a suggested minimum time of one hour per day. Ideally, however, the patient should practice long enough and frequently enough for habituation or new learning to occur.

If you are assigning homework based on an imaginal exposure exercise conducted during the session, you can advise the patient to listen to the recording of the exposure repeatedly for an hour (without interruption per day, but again, ideally long enough and frequently enough for habituation or new learning to occur). You can also instruct the patient to write down any problems or comments she encounters with the assignment, so that they can be reviewed and discussed at the next session (or during the phone contact, if applicable).

### Self-Help Book Assignment (Optional)

If the patient was assigned a self-help book and has already started reading it, you can ask her for a summary of the main points and ask whether she has any questions based on what she has read thus far. Be sure that the patient's understanding of the content is sound before moving on. If she failed to complete the assignment, you can review the rationale for using a self-help book to augment the therapy, assess what got in the way, collaborate with her to determine whether the assignment is worth repeating, and if so, problem-solve to ensure that the assignment will be completed before the next session.

### Item for Ex/RP (Optional)

If the patient was assigned to bring in an item to be used for Ex/RP, be sure to check whether the patient completed this task. If the patient failed to bring in the item, you can review the rationale for selecting the item, assess what got in the way, and collaborate with the patient to problem-solve how to ensure that the item will be brought to a future session.

# BRIEF REVIEW OF THE CBT MODEL OF OCD AND RATIONALE FOR EXPOSURE

Ask the patient to explain the CBT model of OCD and how the model can be used to explain the rationale for Ex/RP. If the patient can do so with minimal or no corrections needed, you can move on to assess the patient's current motivation level to engage in Ex/RP (see the next section). If the patient struggles, you can attempt to determine whether the patient's difficulty is related to a reluctance to do the in-session Ex/RP or whether it is due to a true deficit in understanding the model and rationale for treatment. If the latter, you can briefly review the model and rationale once again, correcting any misunderstandings, and then reassign a review of the handouts and session notes for homework.

# BRIEF CHECK ON THE PATIENT'S MOTIVATION TO ENGAGE IN EX/RP

At this point in the session, it can also be useful to have patients rate their level of motivation (e.g., on a 0–10 point scale) to engage in Ex/RP before actually commencing with it. By having patients rate their level of motivation before each exercise, you can demonstrate (1) how motivation, like all other internal states, can (and will) vary throughout the course of treatment; (2) that they can still engage in Ex/RP even when initially having low motivation (if this is the case); (3) how low motivation may be linked to a focus on negative thoughts/predictions/costs and can be enhanced via cognitive restructuring; (4) how motivation may be inversely related to anxiety; and (5) how motivation can (and will) rise after a successful Ex/RP practice. In Session 5 (the first time doing Ex/RP), this discussion can also be explicitly tied to the discussion that took place in the previous session that was based on a review of the Decisional Balance Worksheet (see Appendix B, Form 2) that the patient had completed for homework.

# BRIEF REMINDER OF THE SESSION STRUCTURE

Explain to the patient that for most of the time remaining in the session, you will focus on doing an exposure exercise, based on the item from the hierarchy that the two of you agreed upon at the end of the previous session, in order to "test out" the CBT model of OCD together. It is important for you to be mindful of the time remaining, so that you can ensure that adequate time remains for habituation and/or new learning to occur. You can normalize any anticipatory anxiety the patient may be feeling while also being careful to avoid providing excessive reassurance about any feared consequences/outcomes; you should advise the patient that it is best just to "take the plunge into the pool" and get started with the exercise. Remind the patient that you are available to assist as a coach, and, when necessary, you will demonstrate how to do the exposure exercise for the patient—especially during the initial phase of the Ex/RP (after which time you should be cautious to prevent the demonstrations from becoming a safety behavior for the patient). Remind the patient that he will be asked to rate the level of his anxiety every few minutes, using the SUDS created during treatment Session 3 (see Chapter 10). Instruct the patient to give his "gut" response as quickly as possible and then refocus on the exercise. You can inform the patient that some time will be left at the end of the session to discuss the results of—and his reactions to—each exposure exercise, as well as to come up with a homework assignment and get feedback on the session. In keeping with the principle of collaborative empiricism, you should ask for the patient's approval of this structure.

# IN-SESSION EX/RP: *IN VIVO* AND/OR IMAGINAL

For patients with particularly severe OCD who elected to have a coach, you should consider with the individual patient whether inviting in the coach at this point might be helpful. This will allow you to model for the coach what a good exposure session looks like and how to be a good coach during exposure. If the patient does not feel comfortable with this idea or if the patient's OCD symptoms are at a more moderate level, it may be more beneficial for you to work alone with the patient during the first few sessions and to consider inviting the coach at a later session, so that the patient can "show off" her skills.

## *In Vivo* Ex/RP

Whenever possible, *in vivo* exposure should be considered the standard exercise for each Ex/RP session. Depending on the type of *in vivo* exposure exercise being conducted, however, it may be implemented in a variety of ways and augmented with cognitive, metacognitive, mindfulness, or acceptance and commitment techniques, based on your conceptualization of the type of learning that needs to occur. As a result, it is important for you to prepare for each session in advance. Regardless of the techniques being used, however, you can always gather the following pieces of information from the patient before the start of each exposure session:

1. Pre-SUDS (anticipatory anxiety)
2. Predicted Max SUDS
3. Feared predictions about the anxiety and/or consequence(s) of engaging in the exposure exercise (assuming ritual prevention will be in effect both during and after the exercise) and strength of belief in them, on a 0–10 scale
4. Typical coping strategies/rituals/safety behaviors (including mental rituals) that the patient will want to use
5. Willingness to prevent the use of these coping strategies/rituals/safety behaviors (including mental rituals), on a 0–10 scale

Based on the above information, you may elect to make the exposure session consist of one long trial (e.g., having a patient with contamination fears keep her hands in contact with a contaminated object for a prolonged period of time) or a series of shorter trials (e.g., walking in and out of rooms while intentionally thinking a forbidden thought). In addition, as noted previously, although it has traditionally been suggested that therapists always allow enough time for habituation to occur, more recent research suggests that it may not be necessary for habituation to occur for gains to be made. There may be instances in which it is more appropriate to intentionally end without habituation occurring (e.g., if the patient believes he will "not be able to function" if he leaves your office feeling anxious).

It is beyond the scope of this book to describe how to set up Ex/RP exercises for every possible variant of OCD. What is important is that you and the patient use the CBT model and case formulation as a guide. In essence, each exposure session can be treated like a scientific experiment, aimed at testing the idiosyncratic model that was created to account for the patient's symptomatology. As such, patients should understand that Ex/RP is simply a method (e.g., enabling one to face a trigger and/or obsession, without using any safety behaviors or rituals) that will allow them to "test" their hypothesis (i.e., challenge their predictions and beliefs) about what will happen—in terms of both how they deal with anxiety and the consequences of their actions (e.g., getting sick). Therefore, it is critical that each exposure be customized to test out a specific fear held by the patient and set up in a way that allows new learning to occur.

Recall that predictions, as in any scientific experiment, need to be operationalized in order to be tested. Therefore, consequences must be made as specific, measurable, and time-limited as possible. For example, patients with obsessions about contamination may state that their fear is that they will "get sick" if they touch your office door handle and then not wash their hands right away, and rate their belief in this as high (e.g., "9/10"). Before conducting the exposure, you should work with the patient to make the prediction as specific as possible, such as by ascertaining (1) whether the length of time without washing after contact would change the odds of the patient becoming ill, (2) how much time would lapse before the patient became ill, (3) what type of illness the patient would contract, and (4) how the patient would know it was because of the particular exposure exercise. In addition, if you will be modeling the exposure exercise for the patient, it is important to ask whether the same predictions apply to you (and if not, why not).

Other patients with obsessions about contamination may instead focus on their anxiety level, rating their belief as high (e.g., "9/10"), indicating that their anxiety level would "continue to rise" or "never come down," eventually making them "go crazy" if they had to touch your door handle without washing their hands afterward. Once again, before conducting the exposure, you should work with the patient to make the prediction as specific as possible. For example, you should ascertain (1) how the two of you will be able to tell if the anxiety level is rising (e.g., which physiological symptoms should be monitored?); (2) how much time would have to elapse before the patient "goes crazy"; and (3) what exactly "going crazy" would mean (the patient should be forced to define the term "crazy"—for example, would the patient then be diagnosed with a new mental disorder?). And once again, if you will be modeling the exposure exercise for the patient, it is important to ask whether the same predictions apply to you (and if not, why not).

With the above examples in mind, while engaging in the exposure, you would want to ensure that the patient touches the door handle—with both hands and with each hand making full contact with the handle (e.g., wrapping the fingers from both hands around the entire door handle). While doing this, content should be made for as long as it takes to activate the patient's thoughts about the consequences of being contaminated, to learn something new about the nature of his anxiety (e.g., that it rises and falls), and/or to test his prediction that his anxiety level would continue to rise and never come down, eventually making him go crazy. It can also be helpful to get a new belief rating from the patient after the exposure. If circumstances make it difficult to maintain continuous contact with the trigger (e.g., the door handle is to a public bathroom), the patient can

can be encouraged to renew contact as soon as possible. Regardless which of the two scenarios (or a combination of both), it is critical to have the patient focus on all of his obsessive thoughts that are occurring in the moment: it is in these moments (increases anxiety) that the patient's fear structure is activated and new learning can occur.

It is also often advisable to encourage patients periodically to "spread the contamination" that they believe is on their hands, all over their body. For example, you can have them rub their hands together (as if "washing" them with the contaminant) and then rub their hands over their clothes, around their head, and all over their face. In addition, if you have been modeling the exposure exercise for the patient, it can be useful for you to "high five" each other (or shake hands) to make sure that whatever contaminant each came in contact with is adequately "spread" to the other (thus ruling out any excuses for why a feared outcome did not occur).

You can do several things during these exposure exercises to maximize their benefit to the patient. For example, at times you may want to (1) normalize any anxiety that the patient may be feeling and explain it as a sign that the two of you are doing things correctly, as the patient has likely been avoiding or ritualizing for some time in order to manage her anxiety and/or feared consequences; (2) offer words of validation and encouragement (while limiting reassurance); (3) express confidence in the model and treatment; (4) observe whether the patient tries to manage her anxiety with any rituals or safety behaviors (overt or covert); (5) ask and note her SUDS level on an Ex/RP Practice Record (see Figure 10.3 in Chapter 10 and Appendix B, Form 10, for a blank copy); (6) ask and note on an Ex/RP Practice Record her level of belief in feared outcomes and/or consequences (from 0 to 10); and/or (7) engage in formal cognitive, metacognitive, mindfulness, or acceptance and commitment techniques (see Chapter 14).

After the exposure is complete, be sure to always gather the following pieces of information from the patient.

1. Post-SUDS anxiety rating
2. Calculation of actual Max SUDS (from ratings obtained during the exercise) and comparison with predicted Max SUDS at the start of the session
3. Results of feared predictions about the anxiety and/or consequence(s) of engaging in the exposure exercise and a new rating of the patient's strength of belief in these predictions, on a 0–10 scale
4. Alternative beliefs about the anxiety and/or consequence(s) and a rating of strength of belief in them from 0–10
5. Any urges to engage in rituals and if present, how strong, on a 0–10 scale
6. Willingness to prevent the use of these coping strategies/rituals/safety behaviors (including mental rituals), on a 0–10 scale

Allow enough time for (1) a discussion of any new learning that took place, (2) feedback from the patient on the exposure exercise, (3) identification of any upcoming challenges (e.g., not washing right after session), (4) the assigning of homework, (5) feedback for you, (6) the patient's summary of the session and take-home message, and (7) any scheduling issues to be clarified.

From Session 6 onward, some time can also be allocated to review any progress the patient has made in either working up the hierarchy or, if necessary, repeatedly facing a particularly challenging item. If the patient mentions feeling frustrated, "stuck," or less motivated, it can be useful to (1) normalize and validate these feelings, (2) discuss the nature of improvement as nonlinear, (3) frame these moments as opportunities and challenges rather than threats, (4) problem-solve (e.g., homework compliance, ritual prevention, hierarchy adjustments), (5) review progress made on previous items, (6) review the Decisional Balance Worksheet (see Appendix B, Form 2) or create a new one, and/or (7) note any ways in which the patient's efforts put in thus far have created a tangible difference in his life.

If a coach is being used but was not invited to participate during the session, it is advisable to have the coach attend the postexposure information-gathering portion of the session. This way the coach can remind the patient between sessions of the new learning that took place and how the patient felt after the exercise, keep the patient focused on ritual prevention after the session, and add his input on any problematic behaviors and/or improvements that he has observed—in either the patient's ability to manage her symptoms and/or function in the world.

Sessions 6 through 14 can be conducted in a manner similar to this session, with the goal being to get to the most challenging items as quickly as possible. As a result, as many of the Ex/RP sessions as possible can be dedicated to helping the patient face his most challenging triggers and problem-solve any roadblocks that may occur along the way. Ideally, you should aim to reach the highest item on the hierarchy with at least two or three sessions left (i.e., by Session 11 or 12), so that the remaining exposure sessions can be used to (1) repeat exercises or slight variations thereof for the most challenging items on the hierarchy (to ensure that the patient's anxiety has been extinguished/significantly diminished/generalized); (2) repeat exposure to any previously faced triggers that have started to generate anxiety again (lapses); or (3) create new exposure exercises for any new triggers that may have emerged that were not included in the original hierarchy.

## Imaginal Ex/RP

As stated earlier in this chapter, whenever possible, *in vivo* exposure should be considered the standard exercise for each Ex/RP session. In some instances, however, the Ex/RP cannot be either ethically or pragmatically carried out *in vivo*. For example, some patients' obsessions involve homicidal, suicidal, or sexually aggressive thoughts. While in these instances you can conduct *in vivo* exposure to some of the triggers (e.g., knives, "vulnerable" subjects), the patient may still report experiencing unwanted thoughts or images of engaging in the actual act. In these cases, it is important for you and the patient to create an imaginal exposure exercise that will allow the patient to face the feared thought or image in a prolonged manner.

As with any *in vivo* exposure exercise, adequate time should be allowed in order for you to (1) provide a rationale for the exposure, (2) structure the exposure exercise in a way that will allow for new learning to take place, and (3) conduct the exercise in collaboration with the patient. In fact, all of the same rules of *in vivo* exposure apply to imaginal exposure—including the gathering of the same pre-exposure information and ratings (see Figure 10.3 for a sample Ex/RP Practice Record and Appendix B, Form 10, for a blank copy), with the sole difference being that in the case of imaginal exposure, the exercise will be done using the patient's imagination.

Often, it is useful to set up the imaginal exposure by having the patient describe the feared scenario in great detail, which you can record—initially in writing (while drafting the scenario) and then using a digital tape recorder (or smart phone voice memo application). Instruct the patient to describe the feared scenario as fully and as vividly as possible, incorporating all of the senses (i.e., what the patient sees, feels, hears) and in the present tense—as if it were happening in the moment. In addition, ensure that the patient does not "neutralize" the scenario in any way (i.e., incorporate details into the scenario that would diminish the patient's level of anxiety and/or prevent a feared outcome from occurring). Finally, it is critical that you customize the imaginal exposure exercise to have the scenario end in a way that maximizes the patient's anxiety. Although this will often involve having the patient imagine encountering a negative outcome that she most feared would happen (e.g., going to jail, ending up in hell, being disowned by family and friends, contracting an illness), at other times, for patients with poor tolerance for uncertainty, it may involve having the patients imagine an outcome in which they never find an answer they are looking for (e.g., whether they have contracted an illness, whether they are practicing their religion appropriately).

Once the imaginal scenario has been drafted, you can have the patient read it over in its entirety, out loud, to make sure that it is complete and anxiety-provoking before considering it final. Once finalized, inform the patient that the goal will be to have the patient read (or recall, with eyes closed, if possible, to maximize the opportunity to filter out distracting stimuli) the imaginal scenario out loud, slowly and deliberately, while trying to picture it as if it were really happening. Remind the patient that he will be asked for a SUDS rating every few minutes (see Figure 10.3 in Chapter 10 for an example) while reading/recalling the scenario, and instruct the patient simply to give his "best guess" rating in that moment, while trying to hold on to the imaginal scene/image, and then return as quickly as possible to describing the scenario. Be sure to check whether the patient has any questions or concerns and be sure to gather same five pieces of pre-exposure information (described above and captured in Ex/RP Practice Record—see Appendix B, Form 10), as in the case of *in vivo* exposure.

As mentioned above, the recording of the imaginal scenario using a digital tape recorder (or smart phone voice memo app) can also be helpful because (1) the patient can take a copy of the scenario home to listen to for homework, (2) it may enhance some patients' ability to "get into" the scenario if they can listen to it rather than read it, and (3) the SUDS ratings given by the patient can serve as a benchmark for measuring progress on the scenario over time (i.e., the ratings reported during taping for the first time should be highest). As is the case with all homework assignments, discuss the importance of listening to the recording for homework (see the homework section, "New Assignments"), and specifically in this case, the risks to confidentiality pertaining to having an electronic file. If necessary in your practice, have the patient sign a release for the recording of the scenario (and any other taped sessions).

Note that, on occasion, some patients report difficulty in visualizing the imaginal scenario and/or that reading/rehearsing it does not evoke much anxiety. In these cases, you can normalize and validate their difficulty and suggest that it may take a few trials before they can really get into the exercise. You can encourage patients to view this as a skill to be practiced, like all of the other skills they have been learning in treatment. In addition, you should be vigilant for subtle ways in which patients may employ safety behaviors—such as by seeking reassurance, asking questions to disengage from reading/rehearsing, editorializing, and/or telling it like it is a story, rather than really imagining themselves being in the situation and describing how they would be feeling if it were really happening.

If, however, after several practice attempts the patient is still unable to generate anxiety by imagining the scene, you may review to ensure that (1) the scenario is vivid enough (i.e., it incorporated all of the senses), (2) the scenario ends with an outcome that the patient believes would be most scary, and (3) no neutralizations are embedded in it. In addition, check to ensure that the scenario is still believable/realistic to the patient (i.e., when crafting the scenario, a balance has been kept between taking it to the worst-case and keeping it within the scope of what the patient believes is possible).

If all of the above measures still fail to make the patient anxious, it may be useful to consider (1) "zooming in" on the scariest part of the scenario (perhaps the detail is allowing the patient to avoid and/or disengage from the feared thought/image), and (2) condensing the scenario down to a single, summary, "worst-case" statement that can be repeated. For example, in some cases, repeating the phrase, "My parents are going to die in a car crash!" (or "My parents may have died in a car crash!") might be more anxiety-provoking than creating an entire scenario in which this happens and the patient finds out about it. The important thing is to be creative and work as a team to find the best method for facing the anxiety-provoking image/thought/scenario.

As with any *in vivo* exposure exercise, after the imaginal exposure is complete, you should always gather postexposure information from the patient (see Ex/RP Practice Record in Appendix B, Form 10). Be sure to also allow enough time for (1) a discussion of any new learning that took place, (2) feedback from the patient on the imaginal exposure exercise, (3) identification of any upcoming challenges (e.g., not ritualizing after the session), (4) assignment of homework, (5) feedback for you, (6) the patient's summary of the session and take-home message, and (7) any scheduling issues to be clarified.

Again, if a coach is being used and was not invited to participate during the imaginal exposure portion of session, it is advisable to have the coach attend the postexposure information-gathering portion of the session, as well as the homework review, rationale, and new assignment portion. This will remind the coach of the importance of the Ex/RP assignments and also remind the patient between sessions of its importance, as well as the new learning that took place and how the patient felt after the exercise, keep the patient focused on ritual prevention after the session, and add his input on any problematic behaviors and/or improvements that he has observed—in either the patient's ability to manage her symptoms and/or function in the world.

## HOMEWORK

### Review of the Rationale (Session 5 Only)

Given that Session 5 will have been the first session of (imaginal or *in vivo*) Ex/RP, it is critical that you reiterate the important role that regular homework/practice plays in determining a positive treatment outcome. You can emphasize that all of the work that has been done up to this point has been to prepare the patient for this challenge. Remind patients that by doing the exposure exercises on their own, without your help, between sessions, they will begin to build the skills needed to face the triggers that currently occur in their lives, as well as any new triggers that may emerge in the future (and thus, prevent relapse down the road).

If mentioned earlier in the treatment, this is the point in time when it can be useful for you to inform patients that this is the "leap of faith" they were warned they would need to take. It is often at this point in the treatment that even the most compliant patients feel a decrease in their motivation to change, struggle with assignments and become noncompliant, and even consider dropping out of therapy. As a result, you should be sure to reinforce the patient for all of the effort she has made up to this point, while also encouraging her to push herself even harder this week, so that she can finally begin to learn something new about her fears and begin to realize all of the benefits she identified in her Decisional Balance Worksheet (see Appendix B, Form 2). Remind the patient to believe in the CBT model and introduce the adage that the "first is the worst" when it comes to facing Ex/RP hierarchy items—as with increased practice, each item will become less anxiety provoking.

If the patient has had issues with homework compliance in previous sessions or seems hesitant about being able to complete the at-home exposure exercise(s) and/or maintain ritual prevention, you can instruct him to focus on taking one step at a time (e.g., take things one hour at a time, if necessary). In addition, you can inform the patient that if he slips (i.e., ritualizes), he should accept that this happens and should recommit to aiming for 100% ritual prevention as soon as possible. You can also remind the patient that if he feels more anxious for the next few weeks, it is a good sign because it means he is now starting to face his fears, after weeks or months or even years of avoiding them—without relying on rituals to feel better.

As always, you should ensure that the patient agrees on the usefulness and importance of the assignments and their connection to her broader goals of treatment. Be sure to suggest that, when in doubt, the patient can review his treatment goal(s) and then commit only to being willing to try to put in the maximum effort he can each day, while accepting that from moment to moment, his motivation (and therefore, success) may vary. Be sure that the patient agrees that engaging in Ex/RP will have a direct impact on his ability to reach his goals. If necessary, you can review the factors that have interfered with the patient's ability to complete the homework in previous sessions and make/adjust a plan with the patient that addresses these obstacles. Finally, you should anticipate with the patient any potential challenges that may arise in the week ahead that may interfere with his ability to successfully complete the homework assignments, and make a plan that addresses these obstacles.

If the patient has enlisted the help of a coach, you can check to see how this arrangement has been working out, and if necessary, remind the coach about how best to be of help to the patient— especially with regard to the patient's exposure practices and ongoing ritual prevention efforts. If you will be acting as a coach to the patient between sessions (i.e., offering phone support between sessions), you can remind the patient about the rules of the phone supports (e.g., frequency, length, and format) and confirm when the next coaching session will occur (e.g., the focus of the call will be on discussing the home-based Ex/RP and problem-solving any slips in ritual prevention).

## New Assignments

As has been the case since the first treatment session, you can have the patient review any notes taken during this session, along with the notes from the previous sessions, and then return with a summary and/or questions. Get a commitment from the patient that she will continue to strive for 100% ritual prevention, especially in the first few hours after leaving your office following each Ex/RP session. Remind the patient that slips should be thought of as learning experiences and recorded on the Self-Monitoring Form (see Appendix B, Form 4), making sure the patient still has enough copies of it.

Give the patient several copies of the Ex/RP Practice Record (see Appendix B, Form 10) and review how to complete it, using the exposure exercise completed in the current session as an example. Instruct the patient to practice Ex/RP each day between sessions, with the exercises targeting the item(s) completed in session, along with any other items from the hierarchy rated at the same SUDS level or below the item from the current session.

You and the patient (and coach, if applicable) should collaborate to agree on which items from the hierarchy the patient will work on for homework. To avoid confusion, it is advisable for you to write these on the Ex/RP Practice Record (see Appendix B, Form 10) as they are agreed upon. You can encourage the patient to practice as much as possible each day, with a suggested minimum time of one hour per day. Ideally, however, the patient should practice long enough and frequently enough for habituation and/or new learning to occur.

If you are assigning homework based on an imaginal exposure exercise conducted during the session, you can advise the patient to listen to the recording of the exposure repeatedly for an hour (without interruption per day but again, ideally long enough and frequently enough for habituation and/or new learning to occur). Be sure to also instruct the patient to write down any problems or comments she encounters with the assignment, so that they can be reviewed and discussed at the next session (or during the phone contact, if applicable).

Finally, before wrapping up each session, you should review with the patient the item planned for the next Ex/RP session and, if the exposure exercise requires an item unique to the patient (e.g., picture of a family member, contaminated object from home), you can remind the patient to bring this in for the next session. Finally, if a self-help book (e.g., *Stop Obsessing!: How to Overcome Your Obsessions and Compulsions* by Edna Foa and Reid Wilson) was assigned to augment the treatment, the patient can be asked to continue reading it to supplement the treatment sessions conducted thus far and to aid his understanding of how the treatment will work from this point on.

## RAPPORT AND ALLIANCE BUILDING: FEEDBACK, SUMMARY, AND TAKE-HOME MESSAGE

As was the case for each of the previous sessions, be sure to continue to build rapport, trust, and a strong working alliance with the patient by eliciting feedback about what was liked and disliked about the session, your performance as a therapist, and how the therapy is progressing. In this way, patients will continue to experience the treatment as a collaborative process and hopefully share more in the responsibility for the treatment outcome. You can also give feedback to the patient about anything positive observed—either in this session or since the initial intake—while also providing constructive, corrective feedback if necessary. In particular, it can be helpful to elicit feedback from the patient on each Ex/RP exercise, the effort the patient anticipates will be required to maintain 100% ritual prevention, the at-home Ex/RP assignment, predictions about the next exposure session, and/or anything else regarding the road ahead (in therapy and beyond).

Finally, you and the patient can take turns (with the patient starting) summarizing the main points of the session, so that you can check the patient's understanding of the materials presented (e.g., the Ex/RP rationale and the conclusions being drawn after the first exposure trial) and in particular the patient's understanding of the main points. If the patient's summary is incomplete or inaccurate, you can add additional thoughts and/or make corrections to the summary, while being sure to check in with the patient to get agreement. Once you and the patient agree on the summary, you can wrap up by once again asking the patient for the take-home message from the session (e.g., "Based on what we covered in our session today, what have you learned and how will this change how you live your life?"). Asking this question reinforces the notion that the material covered in each session is not only important but should also have a practical impact on the patient's life. As a reminder, the summary and take-home message should be logically connected to the homework assignment given for the week to help facilitate transporting the material to outside of the office.

## PREPARING FOR THE HOME VISIT (OPTIONAL)

It is often a good idea to conduct at least one session in the patient's home, near the end of treatment (or earlier, if problems arise regarding compliance with homework) to ensure that the skills learned in therapy generalize into the "patient's world" and that no subtle avoidances/safety behaviors are being performed at home. If a session is going to be used for a home visit, some time should be saved at the end of the session prior to it for home visit preparation. This can include setting an agenda for the visit (including both an in-home assessment of triggers and exposure exercise to be done in the home), rules and expectations (e.g., the patient should treat the appointment like an office appointment, despite it being in the home, dressing appropriately and identifying an appropriate place in the home where the session can be held without interruption), confidentiality (e.g., neighbors, other family members), and who else should be present (e.g., coach, family members, if you will bring a colleague).

---

### TAKE-HOME MESSAGE FROM TREATMENT SESSIONS 5–14

Treatment Sessions 5–14 constitute the core of the treatment: Ex/RP. In so doing, they put to the test the case formulation, as well as all of the hypotheses generated in previous sessions. In an ideal world, you will start these sessions with a highly motivated and hopeful patient who understands the nature of OCD, has a working model of the key perpetuating factors, and a willingness to test out—with your help in session and on her own between sessions—the CBT approach to treating OCD. With a polished hierarchy as a roadmap, these next 10 sessions provide enough time to enable patients to face their most feared triggers (via exposure), while cutting off the rituals that have helped perpetuate the disorder (via ritual prevention). As a result, patients can begin to feel relief almost immediately—as feared consequences do not occur and ritual prevention becomes easier—which will increase their confidence in you, in the treatment model and rationale, and ultimately, in themselves. To ensure this last point, although you and the patient should always work in collaboration, the emphasis on homework assignments and between-session ritual prevention starts to shift the onus of responsibility onto the patient, increasing a sense of mastery and independence, and in turn, a sense of confidence in their ability to manage the symptoms on their own in the future. This principle is further emphasized in treatment Session 15 (the optional home visit).

# CHAPTER 12

# Treatment Session 15

## *The Home Visit*

In some instances a home visit may be impractical or prohibitive due to either distance/travel time for you or a policy (clinic, insurance, associated fees, etc.), and in other instances, it may be unnecessary (e.g., skills have generalized or symptoms not specific to home). On these occasions, session 15 may be used to conduct an additional exposure exercise, provide supplemental strategies (e.g., cognitive, metacognitive, mindfulness, acceptance, etc.), skipped, or combined with session 16 to allow for a more comprehensive relapse prevention component. In the event that a home visit is called for, you should be aware of the additional challenges (safety, confidentiality, etc.) involved in conducting therapy in a patient's home and, as a result, the need to pay added attention and maintain the core elements of the in-office session, such as structure, boundaries, and pacing.

## SESSION COMPONENTS

- Brief check on symptoms
  - Ratings of overall severity of OCD, as well as effort and success at 100% ritual prevention
  - Self-monitoring of OCD symptoms (when unsuccessful at resisting)
  - Optional: Brief check on self-report measure(s)
- Brief review of the homework
  - Notes/summary/questions from the previous session (optional)
  - Between-session *in vivo* and/or imaginal Ex/RP practices
  - Item for in-home Ex/RP
- Brief check on the patient's motivation to engage in Ex/RP
- Brief reminder of the session agenda and structure
- In-home assessment of triggers
- In-home *in vivo* Ex/RP exercise
- Final homework
  - Maintaining momentum using current assignments
  - Repeat in-home *in vivo* Ex/RP plus any remaining items
  - Complete end of treatment questionnaires

- Plan a "slip" (optional)
  - Self-help book assignment (if not already assigned earlier in the treatment)
- Rapport and alliance building: Feedback, summary, and a take-home message
- Preparing for the final session (relapse prevention)


## MATERIALS NEEDED

- Self-report measure(s)
- Writing pad and clip board for you to use
- Copy of the patient's file or last session's note
- Clip board for the patient to take notes during the session
- Item(s) for in-home Ex/RP exercise
- Handouts/forms for homework
  - Self-Monitoring Forms
  - At-home Ex/RP Practice Records
  - End-of-treatment questionnaire packet


## BRIEF CHECK ON SYMPTOMS

Given that this visit takes place in the patient's home, it is important to focus on getting to the in-home assessment of triggers and in-home *in vivo* Ex/RP exercise as quickly as possible. Thus, you and the patient should be sure to select a location to hold the session in the patient's home that minimizes distractions and maximizes confidentiality, set the agenda immediately, and then focus on maintaining the session structure.

As has been the case with the previous Ex/RP sessions, you can ask the patient to rate the overall severity of her OCD, as well as her effort and success at achieving 100% ritual prevention between the sessions, using 0–10 scales. Although in this instance you may not be able to graph the scores, you can offer feedback to the patient on how these numbers compare to her previous scores. Ideally, the patient will have been able to achieve 100% ritual prevention by this point—or will report only the occasional slip. If there have been any slips, normalize them, reinforce any efforts made to complete the monitoring, briefly review and problem-solve these with the patient, and include them in the final homework and/or relapse prevention plan. Encourage the patient to continue monitoring all slips between sessions. Otherwise, you can note any improvements observed and/or reinforce the patient's continued efforts.

### Optional: Brief Check on Self-Report Measure(s)

If the patient has been completing a brief, empirically based, self-report measure of OCD (e.g., the OCI-R; see Appendix C, Form 11) at the start of certain sessions (e.g., weekly, monthly) and is due to complete one at this session, it is advisable to have him complete it at the start of the session, so that you can score it at the start of the session and provide feedback to the patient. As was the case throughout the treatment, it can enhance compliance and motivation if the patient can see objectively that he has made progress (i.e., the score has decreased) and/or be useful for generating a discussion on problem-solving together if treatment stalled (i.e., the score has not changed) or slipped (i.e., the score has increased). If any specific items remain at a level of concern, be sure to discuss these with the patient and include in the final homework and/or relapse prevention plan.

## BRIEF REVIEW OF THE HOMEWORK

### Notes/Summary/Questions from the Previous Session

If the patient took notes or was given any forms or handouts to review between sessions, be sure to briefly check whether she completed these tasks. If so, ask her for a summary of the main points and/or answer any questions or comments she had about them.

### Between-Session *In Vivo* and/or Imaginal Ex/RP Practices

Briefly review the patient's progress on any between-session *in vivo* and/or imaginal Ex/RP assignments. This can be accomplished most efficiently by reviewing the patient's Ex/RP Practice Record (see Figure 10.3 in Chapter 10). Most often, the patient will have been assigned daily Ex/RP practice sessions at home, with or without the aid of the coach (if applicable), with the exercises targeting the item(s) completed in the previous treatment session, along with any other items from the patient's hierarchy that were rated at the same SUDS level or below the item from the most recent session.

If the patient completed the assignment, you can ask her for a summary of how the Ex/RP went, whether any problems were encountered while doing it (or afterward), and any conclusions (i.e., new learning) the patient has drawn. As is the case with all homework assignments, if the patient failed to complete the assignment, you can review the rationale for the assignment, assess what got in the way, and collaborate with her to problem-solve how to ensure that the assignment will be completed before the next session. In addition, in this case, be sure to emphasize the important role that continuing with *in vivo* and/or imaginal Ex/RP assignments in the weeks ahead can have on treatment outcome.

### Item for In-Home Ex/RP

If the patient was assigned to select an in-home item to be used for Ex/RP, you can check whether he completed this task. If the patient completed the assignment, you can praise him but then defer further discussion of item selection until that portion of the agenda (see below). If the patient failed to do so, you can briefly review the rationale for selecting the item and assess what got in the way, but then defer further discussion of item selection until that portion of the agenda (see below).

## BRIEF CHECK ON THE PATIENT'S MOTIVATION TO ENGAGE IN EX/RP

In order to reach this stage of treatment, many patients will have demonstrated a high level of motivation and dedication throughout much of the treatment. Nevertheless, it may be the case that the patient's motivation begins to waiver toward the end of treatment and/or when the treatment setting switches to the patient's home. As a result, it is a good idea to check on the patient's motivation once again, to engage the patient in a brief discussion of the threats to motivation (see Chapter 11), and, if the patient has been rating it prior to the previous Ex/RP sessions, to get a rating of her level of motivation (e.g., on a 0–10 point scale) to engage in Ex/RP again at this point. If the patient's motivation is high, you can praise her while also noting how it still may fluctuate in the future. If the patient's motivation is low, you can examine whether it is linked to any specific negative thoughts/predictions/costs that can be challenged via cognitive restructuring/decisional balance, and the like and also normalize fluctuations in motivation. If necessary, the patient can also be reminded of the discussion that took place earlier in the treatment, and a review of the patient's Decisional Balance Worksheet (see Appendix B, Form 2) can be performed.

## BRIEF REMINDER OF THE SESSION AGENDA AND STRUCTURE

Remind the patient that, as determined at the end of the last session, the remainder of this session will be spent doing a "tour" of the home to assess the level of discomfort caused by any past or present triggers, followed by the *in vivo* Ex/RP exercise that the two of you agreed on last session. Inform the patient that the goal of the home visit is to do a "final test" of the CBT model of OCD together, to see if it can be fully implemented in the patient's life outside of the office (i.e., in the home and beyond). You can normalize any anticipatory anxiety the patient may be experiencing, while being careful to not provide excessive reassurance about any feared consequences/outcomes.

Inform the patient that, as has been the case throughout the treatment, you will be asking him to rate the level of his anxiety every few minutes using the SUDS created earlier in the treatment and instruct him simply to give his "gut response" quickly and then refocus on the exercise. You can also note that, as has been the case for each of the in-office sessions, some time will be saved at the end for processing the Ex/RP, assigning the final homework task(s), as well as getting feedback, a summary, and the take-home message (even though you're at the patient's home this session).

In the spirit of collaboration, be sure to ask for the patient's approval of this structure. For patients who elected to have a coach, you can consider with the patient whether the coach can be invited to join in at this point. Often it is helpful to at least have the coach present while doing the in-home assessment of triggers (past and present). If the patient permits the coach to participate, the coach should be instructed to serve as an observer, unless specifically called on by you or the patient. If the patient does not want the coach to participate at this point, you can suggest that the coach at least be invited to join you at the end of the session so that he or she may be included in the feedback.

## IN-HOME ASSESSMENT OF TRIGGERS

Ask the patient to take you on a "tour" of the home, pointing out objects (e.g., garbage can, stove), areas (e.g., laundry room, bathroom, kitchen), and situations (e.g., leaving the house, entering the bedroom) that are known triggers of her OCD symptoms—both in the past and currently—and getting a current SUDS rating for each of them, along with any factors that may raise or lower her SUDS. Whenever possible, it is advisable to start from outside the front of the patient's home/apartment building. If this step is to be taken, it is useful to make a plan as to how she will handle meeting up with people she may know in the area and what you should or should not say/do. If the patient lives in a house, be sure to include the backyard, garage, and any other areas on the property (e.g., basement, outdoor shed). If the patient lives in an apartment building, be sure to include the parking garage, mailroom, trash room, and so on. If you see a potential trigger that the patient does not point out, be sure to ask about it. Once the tour is complete, be sure to ask if there are any places or triggers that the patient can think of that were skipped and/or any places or triggers that remain challenging. In addition, be sure to ask if the patient has a "safe zone" in the home (e.g., special place protected from contamination).

## IN-HOME *IN VIVO* EX/RP EXERCISE

The in-home Ex/RP exercise can be conducted in the same way that each of the in-office Ex/RP exercises was conducted. Namely, you should be sure to record on an Ex/RP Practice Record (see Appendix B, Form 10) the patient's pre-SUDS rating (anticipatory anxiety), predicted maximum SUDS, feared predictions about the anxiety and/or consequence(s) of engaging in the exposure exercise (assuming ritual prevention will be in effect both during and after the exercise), and strength of belief in it/them from 0 to 10, typical coping strategies/rituals/safety behaviors (including mental rituals) that the patient would typically want to use, and willingness to prevent the use of these coping strategies/rituals/safety behaviors (including mental rituals), from 0 to 10. As is the case with all Ex/RP exercises, be sure to pay particular attention to set up the exposure exercise in such a way as to create the best possible context for new learning to occur—about the patient's anxiety or trigger and/or thoughts (using the case formulation as a guide). Be sure also to operationalize any predictions (i.e., make them specific, measurable, and time-limited) in order to test them out with the patient.

While engaging in at-home Ex/RP, be particularly vigilant to ensure that the patient does not use any safety behaviors or engage in any subtle/partial rituals, for patients often perceive an inflated risk when doing Ex/RP at home. In addition, as mentioned above, patients with severe OCD often have a "safe" place/zone in their homes (e.g., a contamination-free area, such as the bedroom that they have worked hard to "protect" from becoming contaminated). If this is the case, it is critical that you and the patient address this issue but with a heightened sensitivity to the role it has served—often for years.

While conducting the at-home Ex/RP, be sure to act in the same manner as when doing in-office Ex/RP exercises to maximize their benefit to the patient. Namely, you should (1) normalize any anxiety that the patient may be feeling and explain it to be a sign that the two of you are doing things correctly, as he has likely been avoiding and/or ritualizing for some time in order to manage his anxiety and/or feared consequences and now may be confronting the most challenging of triggers in his own home; (2) offer words of validation and encouragement (while limiting reassurance); (3) express confidence in the model and treatment; (4) observe whether the patient tries to manage his anxiety with any rituals or safety behaviors (overt or covert); (5) ask and note on an Ex/RP Practice Record (see Appendix B, Form 10) his SUDS level; (6) ask and note on an Ex/RP Practice Record his level of belief in feared outcomes and/or consequences (from 0 to 10);

and/or (7) engage in formal cognitive, metacognitive, mindfulness, or acceptance and commitment techniques (see Chapter 14).

In-home Ex/RP should also involve recording on the Ex/RP Practice Record the same pieces of information after the exposure exercise has been completed as have been gathered after the in-office Ex/RP exercises. These include (1) obtaining a postexposure SUDS rating; (2) determining the maximum SUDS from ratings obtained during the exercise; (3) reviewing the results of the feared predictions about the anxiety and/or consequence(s) of engaging in the exposure exercise, along with obtaining a new rating of the patient's strength of belief in these predictions using a 0–10 scale; (4) generating alternative beliefs about the anxiety and/or consequence(s) and a rating of strength of belief in these alternative beliefs, from 0 to 10; (5) noting any urges to engage in rituals and, if present, how strong, using a 0–10 scale; and (6) the patient's willingness to prevent the use of these coping strategies/rituals/safety behaviors (including mental rituals), on a 0–10 scale.

As was the case in each of the in-office Ex/RP sessions, be sure also to allow enough time for a discussion of any new learning that took place, feedback from the patient on the exposure exercise (e.g., did the patient note any different experience or outcome by conducting it in the home?) and the identification of any upcoming challenges (e.g., not ritualizing right after session), the assigning of the final homework, feedback on your performance as a therapist, and the patient's summary of the session and take-home message. If the patient has a coach but opted not to include the coach during the tour and/or Ex/RP practice, it is advisable to have the coach attend this portion of the session, so that the coach can remind the patient of the progress made, as well as any new learning that took place and how the patient felt after the exercise. The coach may also help keep the patient focused on ritual prevention after the session. Finally, this will serve as an opportunity to cross-check the in-home assessment of triggers with the coach to ensure the list is complete and the ratings seem accurate.

## FINAL HOMEWORK

Given that this is the first session of in-home Ex/RP as well as likely the last session of Ex/RP that the two of you will do together, it is critical that you highlight the role that continued practice plays in determining successful treatment outcome in the long term. You can emphasize that all of the Ex/RP work completed to this point has been done with the main goal of helping the patient develop the skills necessary for him to use on his own going forward. You can inform the patient that it is important that he be able to do Ex/RP independently, in any context, and be able to apply the skills to any new triggers that may appear in the future. You can note that this idea will be discussed in more detail in the final session, which focuses on relapse prevention.

If there was any indication that the patient struggled more with the in-home Ex/RP than with the in-office Ex/RP, be sure to specifically address how this problem will be approached between sessions (e.g., involve the coach, breaking down challenging items into smaller, less threatening challenges; add cognitive, metacognitive, mindfulness, or acceptance and commitment techniques; review motivational enhancement exercises). In order to maintain momentum, you can then instruct the patient to continue to practice Ex/RP each day between sessions, with a focus on either any difficult areas in the home, any remaining items on the hierarchy, any item(s) on the hierarchy that still evoke more than a minimal level of anxiety, or any new triggers that may emerge. Be sure to reinforce the patient for all of the efforts she has made to date, while also encouraging her to push even more in this, the final week before treatment is terminated. Remind the patient that, when in doubt, she should refer to the CBT model of OCD for guidance on how to approach challenging situations. In addition, you can remind the patient that, much like the first in-office session of Ex/RP you did together, the "first is the worst"—but that with each subsequent practice, the items became less anxiety-provoking. Note, too, that the CBT model of OCD would suggest that this process would be no different when Ex/RP is performed in the home—or anywhere else. You should ensure that the patient has enough copies of the Ex/RP Practice Record (see Appendix B, Form 10) and be sure to copy the results of the Ex/RP exercise that was just completed onto this form to serve as a reminder of how things went. Remind the patient to practice long enough and frequently enough in order for habituation and/or new learning to occur.

Remind the patient to continue to strive for 100% ritual prevention, especially in the first few hours after following the Ex/RP session and encourage the patient, if necessary, to record any "slips" in ritual prevention efforts on the Self-Monitoring Form (see Appendix B, Form 4). In addition, at this point you can ask the patient to generate ideas about how to "undo" any slips in ritual prevention, if they occur (i.e., coming up with an "antiritual" ritual).

Finally, you can provide the patient with any end-of-treatment questionnaires you'd like completed (see Appendix A for a list) and instruct the patient to bring them to the final session. Often it is a good idea to readminister the entire packet used at the start of treatment so that all areas of change (and lack thereof) can be examined and noted. If possible, it is advisable to have the patient drop them off, mail or fax them, or scan and e-mail them ahead of the last session, so that you can score them, and then summarize/provide feedback to the patient during the last session.

## Plan a "Slip" (Optional)

For patients who have progressed steadily throughout the treatment without any major setbacks and who may report that their gains have been due to "luck" or to the fact that they experienced the treatment during a relatively stress-free time, you may want to consider adding a planned "slip" to the final homework. In planning a slip, patients are encouraged to engage in rituals again, for a specific and focused period of time, to observe the impact that this has on them. They should then process what they experienced (e.g., write in a journal about it), including how they coped, what they learned about their OCD, and how they can use this information to help them in the future.

Some patients may report feeling anxious about trying this assignment, which may indicate content missed during the treatment, a lack of confidence in their ability to control the OCD, or the presence of maladaptive cognitions pertaining to the situations, triggers, thoughts, or emotions related to their OCD. In these cases, the rationale can be provided (e.g., it's a good idea to see how you'll handle a slip now, while we're still meeting, so we can discuss how it went and problem-solve any difficulties that arose—and like any other type of exposure, this is yet another instance of helping you build a tolerance for uncertainty). If necessary, these patients can be invited to use the aid of their coach.

## Self-Help Book Assignment (If Not Already Assigned Earlier in the Treatment)

If the patient was not required to purchase and use a self-help book (e.g., *Stop Obsessing!: How to Overcome Your Obsessions and Compulsions* by Edna Foa and Reid Wilson) during the treatment to augment the work, consider recommending one that the patient can purchase to supplement the notes taken during the treatment, for additional psychoeducational material, and/or to enable the patient to further refine her skills by trying to follow the instructions in the book to create her own treatment plan.

## RAPPORT AND ALLIANCE BUILDING: FEEDBACK, SUMMARY, AND A TAKE-HOME MESSAGE

As was the case at the end of each session throughout the treatment, be sure to continue to foster rapport, trust, and a strong working alliance with the patient by eliciting feedback about what he liked and disliked about the session, your performance as the therapist, and how the therapy has progressed. In this way, the patient will continue to experience the treatment as a collaborative process and be more likely to share the responsibility for the treatment outcome. Be sure also to give feedback to the patient about anything positive you observed—either in this in-home session or over the course of therapy—while also providing constructive, corrective feedback if necessary. In particular, it can be helpful to elicit feedback from the patient on how it felt to do the session in her home, her reactions to the in-home assessment of triggers, and how she feels about the fact that the next session will be your last together. The patient can also be asked about the typical end-of-session items, such as the effort the patient anticipates will be required to maintain 100% ritual prevention, repeating the at-home Ex/RP assignment, predictions about the planned slip, or anything else regarding the road ahead—to the last session and beyond.

Finally, you and the patient can take turns (with the patient starting) summarizing the main points of the session, so that you can check her understanding of what happened during this in-home Ex/RP trial. If the patient's summary is incomplete or inaccurate, you can add additional thoughts and/or make corrections to her summary before leaving, while also being sure to check in with the patient to get agreement. Once you and the patient agree on the summary, you can wrap up by once again asking the patient for the take-home message from the session (e.g., "Based on what we covered in our session today, what have you learned and how will this change how you live your life?"). Asking this question reinforces the notion that the material covered in each session is not only important but can also have a practical impact on the patient's life—especially this in-home visit. As a reminder, the summary and take home message should be logically connected to the homework assignment given for the week to help facilitate transporting the material to outside of the office. Finally, if applicable, you can schedule a final phone contact and instruct the patient that the focus of the call will be on discussing the final Ex/RP exercise(s), difficulties completing the final questionnaire packet, and any issues with the planned slip.

## PREPARING FOR THE FINAL SESSION (RELAPSE PREVENTION)

Since the next session will be your last, it is often a good idea to save some time at the end of the session prior to it to prepare for termination. This can include setting an agenda for the last visit (e.g., making a very brief check on symptoms and homework, outlining formal strategies for relapse prevention, processing the end of the therapeutic relationship, and planning for the future) and determining who should be present for it (e.g., coach, family members).

## TAKE-HOME MESSAGE FROM TREATMENT SESSION 15

Treatment Session 15 (if conducted in the home) is used to facilitate the generalization of the skills learned in treatment to the patient's "real world" outside of your office. This is done by ensuring that the patient (and potentially, the patient's coach) is aware of all possible triggers in the home (past and present), is not avoiding, protecting, or treating as special, any areas in the home, and has an opportunity to practice Ex/RP in the home with your guidance. In so doing, the patient is able to experience the same results as in the office: the habituation to anxiety and/or correction of maladaptive beliefs/predictions. The patient therefore continues to learn new information about his OCD symptoms and the treatment while experiencing increased confidence in the model, the treatment, and his ability to manage his symptoms in the real world, should the need arise. As a result, the patient can feel more comfortable with the fact that the treatment will be terminated at the next session.

---
CHAPTER 13
---

# Treatment Session 16

## *Relapse Prevention*

### SESSION COMPONENTS

- Final check on symptoms
  - Optional: Final administration and feedback on self-report measure(s)
- Final review of the homework
  - Ratings of effort and success at 100% ritual prevention and self-monitoring of OCD symptoms (triggers, obsessions, anxiety level, and whether successful at preventing rituals)
  - Generation of ideas about how to undo slips in the future
  - Notes/handouts/questions from the previous session (optional)
  - Report on repeated in-home *in vivo* Ex/RP and/or any new/remaining items
  - Report on planned slip (optional)
  - Collect end-of-treatment packet (if not sent in ahead of the session)
- Final ratings of original exposure hierarchy
- Discuss relapse prevention
  - Conduct a final review of the CBT model of OCD and the rationale for treatment
  - Differentiate a lapse from a relapse
  - Discuss the importance of continuing to use the skills learned in treatment
  - Identify any upcoming high-risk situations
  - Plan to fill in the time freed up by the decrease in symptoms
  - Tapering of ritual prevention and creation of guidelines for "normal" behavior
- Final homework
  - Review notes and handouts from all sessions regularly
  - Begin tapering of ritual prevention and implementation of "normal" behaviors. Continue Ex/RP on any remaining hierarchy items still generating more than mild anxiety and naturalistically on any new items that emerge in the weeks ahead
  - Note signs of lapse and high-risk situations
  - Begin plan to fill in time freed up by decrease in symptoms
  - Self-help book assignment

- Optional: Plan "booster" session
- Rapport and alliance building: Feedback, summary, and a take-home message

## MATERIALS NEEDED

- Self-report measure(s)
- Dry-erase board, easel, or clip board for you to use
- Clip board for the patient to take notes during the session
- Copy of the original finalized hierarchy (for final ratings)
- Handouts/forms for homework
  - Self-monitoring forms
  - At-home Ex/RP Practice Records
  - Self-help book recommendations (optional)

## FINAL CHECK ON SYMPTOMS

It is useful for the patient to give one last subjective report on her effort and success at achieving 100% ritual prevention between sessions (using 0–10 scales), as well as her overall OCD severity. As has been the case throughout the treatment, ideally, these scores will be immediately entered into a chart and a spreadsheet program where they can be graphed; then a final graph can be printed and presented to the patient, so that she can see a summary of how she progressed. You and the patient can examine the graph together and note any patterns between the amount of effort put into ritual prevention, the level of success at ritual prevention, and the overall OCD severity. Ideally, a pattern emerged over time, with effort being higher than success initially, but then reversing over time, and if so, OCD severity decreasing as well. If this is the case, as in all previous sessions, you can reinforce the patient for any improvements observed or normalize any plateaus and/or slips in the treatment progress, and then reframe them as tests of the patient's skills and resolve and as reminders of the need to continue to work hard every day in order to maintain gains. If necessary, you can problem-solve with the patient (e.g., assess level of motivation and insight, homework compliance, comorbidity issues, psychosocial stressor changes).

### Optional: Final Administration and Feedback on Self–Report Measure(s)

If the patient has been completing a brief, empirically based, self-report measure of OCD (e.g., the OCI-R; see Appendix C, Form 11) at the start of certain sessions (e.g., weekly, monthly), it is advisable to have him complete it one last time at the start of this session and then score it (and graph, if possible) immediately. If graphing the results, you can print a final copy for the patient and provide feedback on the results, noting any changes in the scores over time. If any specific items remain at a level of concern, be sure to include a plan for how they will be addressed in the final homework/relapse prevention plan. As in previous sessions, it can enhance motivation to continue to use the skills after termination if the patient (1) can see objectively that progress was made, (2) understand that variations in symptoms are normal, and (3) has a specific plan on how to address any remaining areas of difficulty after treatment has ended.

# FINAL REVIEW OF THE HOMEWORK

## Ratings of Effort and Success at 100% Ritual Prevention and Self-Monitoring of OCD Symptoms

Ask if the patient engaged in any rituals since the last session (home visit). Ideally, the patient will now have been able to achieve 100% ritual prevention since the last session—or will report having had only an occasional slip. If there have not been any slips, you can ask if the patient experienced any urges to ritualize since the last session and, if so, how they were prevented. You can also reinforce the success the patient had in preventing them and then encourage the patient to continue monitoring any slips in the future. If there have been some slips (other than the planned slip—see below), you can normalize them, reinforce any efforts the patient made to complete the monitoring, and briefly review the entries completed by the patient on the Self-Monitoring Form (see Appendix B, Form 4; to determine if any new triggers or symptoms emerged that were not previously mentioned). You can then encourage the patient to continue monitoring any slips in the future and you can problem-solve with the patient how this will be done.

## Generation of Ideas about How to Undo Slips in the Future

Regardless of whether or not the patient was 100% successful at preventing rituals between sessions, be sure to ask the patient what ideas she has about ways to "undo" any slips that may occur in the future. For example, a patient with concerns about contamination may be encouraged to carry around a "contamination" cloth (a cloth that has touched "contaminated" objects), so that any ritualized washing or cleaning can be "undone" by re-contaminating with the cloth. As another example, a patient with checking rituals who slipped (e.g., checked that the oven knob was really set to "off") can be encouraged to turn the dial on and off again quickly and then walk away without checking again.

## Notes/Handouts/Questions from the Previous Session (Optional)

If the patient took notes or was given any forms or handouts to review between sessions, you can briefly check whether he completed these tasks; if so, ask him for a summary of the main points and/or answer any questions or comments he had about them.

## Report on Repeated In-Home *In Vivo* Ex/RP and/or Any New/Remaining Items

Ask if the patient experienced any difficulties in completing the exposure homework (repeating in-home *in vivo* Ex/RP and/or any new/remaining items). If so, ask how she dealt with them and how she plans to remedy similar challenges that may arise after the treatment has ended.

## Report on Planned Slip (Optional)

If the patient was assigned a planned "slip" for homework, be sure to ask him for a report on which rituals he chose to engage in, for how long, and in what context. You can also ask how the patient felt before, during, and after performing the rituals, how he coped, what he learned about his OCD, how he can use this information to help himself in the future, and for any other observations the patient made (ideally in writing). Finally, if the patient had the option of using the aid of his coach, you can ask how this went—and if in fact the coach was used.

### Collect End-of-Treatment Packet (If Not Sent in Ahead of the Session)

If the patient completed and sent in the end-of-treatment questionnaire packet ahead of this session, it is advisable for you to have scored them and to be prepared to discuss a summary of the results. Often the results can best be presented using a table that lists each measure, along with the pre- and posttreatment scores and any clinical interpretations (e.g., mild, moderate, severe). If the patient did not complete and send in the end-of-treatment questionnaire packet ahead of time, you can collect the packet at this point and then consider either sending the patient a summary in the future or presenting a summary of the results in the (optional) "booster session" (see below). If the patient did not complete the packet at all, you can review the rationale for the assignment, assess what got in the way, and then collaborate with the patient to problem-solve how to ensure that the packet gets completed (e.g., the patient may be encouraged to remain after the session to complete the packet or to complete the packet for homework and then return it to you as soon as possible).

## FINAL RATINGS OF ORIGINAL EXPOSURE HIERARCHY

Regardless of whether the patient's exposure items and their respective SUDS ratings were recorded on the Hierarchy Construction Worksheet (see Appendix B, Form 9) or in an electronic database such as a Microsoft Excel spreadsheet, be sure to either have the file open or have printed a copy of the final hierarchy, with an additional column added at the end—either beside the column with the original ratings or after the latest update, if updates were performed throughout the treatment (see Figure 13.1). Inform the patient that the goal is to review the items one last time and get a final set of ratings for each item. Be sure to get the final ratings without first discussing/showing the patient the original ratings (or any of the updates). Instruct the patient to rate each item on the hierarchy based on how anxious she would feel if she had to face it *today* (i.e., "What would your SUDS be for [item X] today?"). Start at the bottom item of the hierarchy and then work up to the most challenging item (as originally rated). Ideally, the SUDS of all of the items will have decreased to only mild/minimal levels. If this is the case, be sure to note these drops in the ratings and, if possible, enter them into the database so that a final copy of the hierarchy, with the pre- and posttreatment ratings can be given to the patient. As mentioned above, it can enhance the patient's motivation to continue to practice the skills learned after treatment has terminated if the patient can see how much progress was made. If any items on the hierarchy were rated at more than a mild/minimal SUDS level (i.e., more than 1–2/10), be sure to discuss and then collaborate with the patient to problem-solve how to ensure that these items are addressed in the final homework/relapse prevention plan.

| Item | Initial SUDS (Date: 1/1/16) | Final SUDS (Date: 5/1/16) |
|---|---|---|
| Using public toilet | 100 | 50 |
| Touching floor (busy area) | 99 | 40 |
| Touching bathroom door handle (inside) | 95 | 30 |
| Touching bathroom faucet handles | 90 | 25 |
| Touching urinal handle | 85 | 20 |
| Touching inside of garbage can | 80 | 25 |
| Lying down on office floor | 75 | 0 |
| Touching seat cushion on public chair | 70 | 0 |
| Handling money | 70 | 5 |
| Touching bathroom door handle (outer) | 65 | 10 |
| Touching office door knob | 60 | 0 |
| Using public telephone | 55 | 20 |
| Touching outside of garbage can | 50 | 0 |
| Touching keyboard | 50 | 15 |
| Touching seatback on public chair | 45 | 0 |
| Touching elevator buttons | 45 | 10 |
| Touching light switch | 40 | 0 |
| Touching floor (corner of room) | 30 | 0 |

**FIGURE 13.1.** Sample Hierarchy Construction Worksheet from treatment Session 16.

## DISCUSS RELAPSE PREVENTION

The bulk of the remainder of the session should focus on discussing relapse prevention strategies with the patient. Although this can be accomplished in a variety of ways, in keeping with the style of previous sessions, it is best to try to do so in a Socratic and interactive style. In this way you can assess how much of the theory, model, and treatment rationale the patient has grasped and ask questions, when necessary to help correct any misunderstandings or gaps in the patient's knowledge. For patients using a coach, it is advisable to have the coach attend this portion of the session, so that you can ensure that the patient has appropriate support and guidance after treatment ends and, in so doing, maximizes the resources available to prevent a relapse from occurring in the future.

## Conduct a Final Review of the CBT Model of OCD and the Rationale for Treatment

The relapse prevention discussion should start with a final review of the CBT model of OCD as well as the rationale for treatment. You may choose to do this by conducting a brief role play in which you (or the patient's coach, if applicable) takes on the role of a patient who has been diagnosed with OCD and the patient now must explain the CBT model of OCD and rationale for the treatment to you (or the coach). Alternatively, you may choose to conduct a brief "quiz" on the topics. Either way, it is important for you to try not to jump in too early/often with corrections and instead allow the patient adequate time to come up with the answers on his own. You should also strive to ascertain if the patient can demonstrate a general understanding of the core principles, rather than getting caught up on specific wording or terms (unless doing so would help clarify whether he truly understands the model and/or rationale). At this point, it would also be appropriate to play a slightly more challenging patient in the role play. At the same time, remember that the goal is to reinforce the patient for demonstrating a general understanding of the model and rationale, and how he can refer to these in the future to prevent a relapse from occurring.

## Differentiate a Lapse from a Relapse

Next, define and differentiate a *lapse* from a *relapse*. You may want to begin by asking the patient if he is able to distinguish between the two. If the patient struggles with this question, inform him that the OCD symptoms, though greatly reduced, will likely still fluctuate in severity over time and, as such, if and when they flare up, they should be seen as a *lapse* (i.e., a temporary change from the current state and/or direction of progress). A *relapse*, however, should be defined as a *full return to a previous (baseline) state and/or level of functioning*. The important thing to highlight here is that *at the moment in time in which a change occurs, it is impossible to determine whether it is a lapse or a relapse*. Therefore, what ultimately distinguishes the two terms ends up being what happens *after* the flare-up. Encourage the patient to consider what people can think, do, and feel after experiencing a flare-up of symptoms (i.e., "slip") that would turn it into a *lapse* (e.g., patients who lapse think of it as just a slip, treat it as an opportunity to learn something new about their triggers and responses, don't beat themselves up about it, and take steps to get back on course again). Next, encourage the patient to consider what people can think, do, and feel after experiencing a change/ slip that would turn it into a *relapse* (e.g., patients who relapse think of it as a sign that they have failed, become depressed or anxious, generate faulty beliefs about themselves, the treatment, and their future, stop using the skills that had been working for them, and return to engaging in the maladaptive behaviors they used to perform prior to starting treatment).

## Discuss the Importance of Continuing to Use the Skills Learned in Treatment

Next, you can note that treatment outcome data suggest that, in general, patients who are followed after treatment ends can (1) maintain their gains, (2) see continued improvement, or (3) witness a deterioration in their gains made in treatment. Ask the patient to consider the factors that determine the different patterns of outcome. In general, you should be looking to see if the patient understands the importance of staying motivated to continue using the skills used in treatment and/or using the concepts learned when facing any new triggers (or old ones that return).

## Identify Any Upcoming High-Risk Situations

Discuss the importance of being able to anticipate any potentially stressful situations that may trigger a return of symptoms and having a plan in place in advance for how to deal with them. With this in mind, you and the patient can look ahead in the patient's calendar and identify any potential stressful situations and label these as "high-risk" or "red-flag" situations. Once identified, you and the patient can begin to construct a plan for how to the patient can prepare for them before being confronted with them. Often, input from the patient's coach can be helpful here—either in recalling past stressors that may cycle back into the patient's life or in anticipating upcoming stressors that the patient may not have considered.

## Plan to Fill in the Time Freed Up by the Decrease in Symptoms

With the gradual but steady decrease in symptoms over the course of treatment, many patients are suddenly left with large blocks of time that were previously spent occupied obsessing and/or engaging in rituals. In addition, there may be many areas or situations in the patient's life that the patient had either previously avoided in order to manage her OCD symptoms or had simply been unable to cope with due to the intensity of the symptoms (e.g., working, dating, socializing). You can examine the amount of time the patient now has free and make a plan with the patient on how it will be filled. You can encourage the patient to consider the things she values most (e.g., friendships, family relations, dating/intimate relations, parenting, faith, physical well-being, recreation, education) and to invest the time that has now been freed up by reducing the OCD into these areas (after prioritizing them). Help the patient to set specific goals to strive toward and to generate a plan involving small steps to be performed on a daily basis that move her toward the goal(s). If major areas of life have been cast aside because of the OCD (e.g., work, interpersonal relationships), consider referring the patient for additional services or assign additional self-help books.

## Tapering of Ritual Prevention and Creation of Guidelines for "Normal" Behavior

Remind the patient that it is normal to experience OCD symptoms and that it only crosses over into being a disorder when the symptoms of OCD take up a great deal of time or cause significant distress or impairment. Therefore, as nearly everyone experiences some of the symptoms of OCD throughout their lives, it is also likely that the patient will continue to experience some OCD symptoms, which will likely fluctuate in severity over time, after the treatment ends. As many patients may have suffered from OCD for many years, however, it may be difficult for them to differentiate what is *normal* from what is *OCD*. As a result, they may struggle initially when loosening up the ritual prevention requirements and may have difficulty determining guidelines for how to act like people without the disorder (i.e., like "normal" people).

It is therefore important for you and the patient to construct a "tapering schedule" for the ritual prevention requirements that were put into place during the treatment and then to create a set of guidelines (note: not rigid rules) for what "OCD-like" behaviors the patient should consider to be "normal" in the weeks and months following the termination of treatment. For example, the guiding questions for normal behavior might be, "What does the typical person without OCD do in this situation?" and "Should I act the same way, given my history with the disorder?"

In general, the tapering of ritual prevention is best done slowly and gradually. For example, you might propose a tapering schedule that allows a gradual return/increase in frequency of behaviors previously banned/limited (e.g., hand washing, cleaning, checking, counting), week by week, over a few weeks. When establishing guidelines on what behaviors should be considered normal going forward, be sure to emphasize to the patient that, at least initially, it is best to err on the side of being conservative (i.e., when in doubt about whether a behavior is appropriate, assume that OCD could be playing a role). One helpful guideline is to have patients consider whether *anxiety* is driving their behavior (in which case it may be a ritual) versus *preference* (in which case OCD is less likely). Ideally, this entire process, like all other aspects of the treatment, should be done collaboratively with the patient.

## FINAL HOMEWORK

In the spirit of fostering greater independence, you can have the patient set her own homework for the future. Ideally, this will incorporate information from the discussion on relapse prevention (see above) as well as include all of the typical items, such as regularly reviewing notes and handouts from all sessions; beginning the tapering of ritual prevention and implementation of "normal" behavior; continuing Ex/RP on any remaining hierarchy items still generating more than mild anxiety and "naturalistically" as new triggers emerge and/or old triggers return; keeping note of any potential high-risk situations and reviewing signs of a lapse; taking the first steps to fill in the time freed up by a decrease in symptoms; and reading a self-help book (if necessary). For patients using a coach, consider having the patient set up an "appointment" with the coach (e.g., as if it is a session with you) to review the assignments. For patients without a coach, you can encourage them to create "appointments" with the same frequency and duration that the two of you met, for the next few weeks, to ensure they set aside some time to continue to practice their skills.

## OPTIONAL: PLAN "BOOSTER" SESSION

For patients who (1) presented with severe OCD, (2) struggled with assignments and/or concepts, (3) continue to experience symptoms late in the treatment, (4) report feeling anxious about terminating, and/or (5) appear to be at particularly high risk of relapse, you may want to schedule a "booster" session. This is typically scheduled anywhere from 2 to 4 weeks after this last session, with the idea that the patient will continue to work on his own (or with the help of the coach, if using one), and then return for a "check-up" to see how things are progressing and problem-solve any difficulties encountered after treatment ended. The session structure would be similar to this relapse prevention session.

Many patients find this more gradual disconnection from therapy to be more tolerable, for it gives them more of a chance to practice the skills and develop confidence in their ability to manage their OCD symptoms on their own, while still having a "safety net" under them (i.e., knowing they will be seeing you at least one more time). This also allows you to check on the progress of the patient and identify and correct any slips or problems that may have occurred while they are still relatively simple and easy to address. It also can serve as an incentive for patients to keep practicing the skills, as they know they will be accountable to you in the future—for the work they've done as well as how they've been managing their symptoms.

If utilized and found to be helpful, you and the patient may choose to continue to arrange for additional booster sessions, often with increasing time between them (e.g., the first at one month, the second at two months after the first, and the third at three months after the second) to keep momentum going and facilitate a smooth transition into independence for the patient. In addition, these may be best if "scheduled in pencil" meaning that if things are going well and the patient feels confident in her ability to manage things on her own, the session, with appropriate notice, can be canceled and rescheduled for a later time.

## RAPPORT AND ALLIANCE BUILDING: FEEDBACK, SUMMARY, AND A TAKE-HOME MESSAGE

As was the case at the end of each session throughout the treatment, be sure to save some time at the end of the session for processing. Even at the last session, you can continue to foster rapport, trust, and a strong working alliance with the patient by eliciting feedback about what he liked and disliked. Only now the focus may be not just on the session, but on the entire treatment, and the role you played along the way. Be sure to give feedback to the patient about anything positive observed—either in this session or over the course of therapy—while also providing constructive, corrective feedback if necessary. In particular, be careful to deflect any attempts by the patient to attribute success only to you; instead, reinforce the notion that it was a *collaborative* effort and in fact that it was the patient who had to do the "heavy lifting" along the way. It can also be useful for you to elicit feedback from the patient about how it feels to be ending treatment and to share your own feelings about the treatment being over.

You and the patient can then take turns (with the patient starting) at summarizing not just the main points of the session but also the main points, skills taught, and lessons learned throughout the therapy. This will allow you and the patient to review all of the work that was accomplished together and the tools available for the patient's use in the future. If the patient's summary is incomplete or inaccurate, you can add additional thoughts and/or skills taught and lessons learned throughout the therapy. It is often helpful if the patient writes these out for review in the future.

Finally, you can wrap up by once again asking the patient for her take-home message—only this time not only from the session, but from the entire treatment (e.g., "Based on what we accomplished in therapy, what have you learned and how will this change how you live your life?"). Asking this question reinforces the notion that all of the material covered was done so with intention and planning to prepare the patient for this moment and to give the patient the skills necessary to manage her OCD symptoms in the future.

# TAKE-HOME MESSAGE FROM TREATMENT SESSION 16

Treatment Session 16 focuses on terminating the therapy and setting the patient up for success in the future (i.e., relapse prevention). This is accomplished by first performing final checks on the patient's symptoms and ability to manage them—including all items on the hierarchy as well as the planned slip (if assigned)—as well as the patient's understanding of the CBT model for OCD and treatment rationale for Ex/RP. The session then transitions to the future by examining collaboratively the patient's plan for continuing Ex/RP on any remaining hierarchy items still generating more than mild anxiety and naturalistically on any new items that emerge in the weeks ahead, and the patient's ability to understand how to anticipate high-risk situations, deal with lapses using the skills learned in treatment, taper off from ritual prevention, engage in normal behavior, and plan for filling the time freed up by a reduction in the OCD symptoms. It also allows you and the patient time to process the ending of the treatment and therapeutic relationship, while offering flexibility in creating booster sessions for those patients who need a more gradual termination.

# CHAPTER 14

# Supplementary Techniques

As is illustrated throughout this book, the core of this treatment planner involves engaging patients in Ex/RP, which various expert consensus guidelines consider to be the "gold-standard" psychological treatment for patients with OCD (see Appendix A). When conducted properly, Ex/RP can be a powerful and robust psychological intervention that can help many patients experience a marked reduction in their symptoms and, as such, reduce disability and dysfunction, helping patients to achieve a vast improvement in their quality of life.

As noted previously, however, you should be careful to *customize the treatment to fit the particular needs of the patient* (i.e., be "personalistic"), rather than try to *force the patient to fit the therapy* (i.e., be "procrustean"). In other words, you should begin treatment with a customized plan that suits each individual patient's circumstances and diagnosis/diagnoses, with the understanding that, at various times throughout the treatment, the case formulation and treatment plan will likely have to be adjusted as new data are obtained from both the patient and from assessment of how the therapy is working. Logically then, you must be willing to consider adjusting the treatment goals, the pacing of the treatment, and even the techniques being used, in order to address each patient's specific needs and life circumstances.

For example, as expert consensus guidelines suggest beginning treatment of OCD with either CBT alone or a combination of CBT and a medication, if you are not licensed to prescribe medications, you may want to consider making a referral to a psychiatrist for a medication evaluation. And if medications are indeed warranted and prescribed, you should account for the role that medication(s) will play in the treatment when generating the case formulation and treatment plan. Similarly, if the patient is already taking medication(s) at intake, it is important that you consider their potential impact (positive and negative) on the symptoms and course of therapy when creating and implementing the treatment plan—and whether you would want to advocate tapering off of the medication(s) at some point during the treatment.

In addition to Ex/RP and medications, expert consensus guidelines suggest that a number of other psychological techniques and interventions can benefit patients diagnosed with OCD. For example, as mentioned earlier in this book, the *cognitive model* of OCD places a greater emphasis on the key role that faulty appraisals play in perpetuating the symptoms of the disorder. As such, a number of specific *cognitive techniques* have been created and tested in the treatment of OCD, which in this case can be used to augment the Ex/RP.

As a result, this chapter will describe examples of several cognitive techniques, as well as some techniques derived from several other psychological approaches (e.g., acceptance and commitment therapy and metacognitive therapy). All of these techniques have some empirical support in the treatment of OCD but without necessarily as many trials completed as Ex/RP. If there is one theme unifying all of these additional approaches, it seems to be that patients are encouraged to *develop a new relationship with their thoughts* (e.g., by instead examining appraisals or by being mindful of thoughts and/or detaching or "defusing" from thoughts and/or accepting them).

All of these approaches are designed to be *optional* components in this treatment planner. As such, they may be excluded altogether if treatment with Ex/RP is progressing steadily, or they may be included, in any order, with or without adaptation, prior to commencing Ex/RP, while engaging the patient in Ex/RP, or after completing a course of Ex/RP. As always, the decision of whether to include these techniques, and if so, which ones to include and when to include them, will depend on your ever-evolving case conceptualization of the patient's OCD and assessment (subjective and/or objective) of how successfully the therapy is unfolding.

## COGNITIVE THERAPY TECHNIQUES

Cognitive models of OCD stress the importance of pathological cognitive processes in the development of the disorder, with the assumption being that these pathological cognitive processes involve evaluative processes linking the obsession and the compulsion (van Oppen & Arntz, 1994). In particular, cognitive models propose that two main evaluative processes take place in OCD: the *perception of threat/danger* and the *appraisal of personal responsibility*. In other words, when patients with OCD believe they must do something to prevent or reduce a perceived danger and/or their perceived personal responsibility, they will feel an increase in distress, which will eventually drive them to perform a compulsion. Therefore, cognitive therapy techniques for OCD generally aim to modify the distress associated with the obsessions (and, in so doing, the urge to neutralize or undo them by performing a compulsion or ritual), primarily by challenging overestimated appraisals of threat/danger and perceptions of inflated personal responsibility. This can be accomplished in a variety of ways, which are described next.

### Cognitive Techniques to Challenge the Overestimation of Threat/Danger

In order to successfully challenge overestimations of threat/danger, you must be sure to address the two components that are hypothesized to inflate the patient's sense of threat/danger: (1) overestimations of the *likelihood* of something bad happening (e.g., "If I touch that handrail, then I'll contract a disease!" or "If I don't lock my car doors, then someone will break into my car!"); and (2) overestimations of the *severity of the consequences* (e.g., "If I get a cold sore, it will get infected and my face will become physically deformed!" or "If I have yogurt in my fridge that is past the expiry date and someone eats it, they will get food poisoning and die!"). An oft-used formula in the literature to describe this appraisal type is: risk = likelihood × severity of consequences. This formula is important to keep in mind, as it represents the notion that perceived risk (i.e., threat or danger) will remain high even when the likelihood of an event is seen as low, if the severity of the consequences of the event is seen as high. Thus, both the likelihood and the severity of consequences will likely need to be addressed to reduce the patient's appraisal of risk/threat/danger.

Overestimations of the *likelihood* of something bad happening can be addressed using various cognitive techniques, the most common of which is to perform a calculation of the probability of the feared outcome happening. The patient should first be asked to state how likely he feels that the outcome would occur, by giving a percentage ranging from 0% (not at all likely) to 100% (definite). This estimation is then compared with an estimation of the likelihood that is based on an analysis of the *sequence of events* that would need to occur in order for the feared outcome to take place. To complete this step, you and the patient first generate the sequence of events that the patient believes would lead to the feared outcome. You then ask the patient to estimate the chance of *each event* in the sequence separately. Finally, you and the patient calculate the *cumulative probability*, which is then compared with the *original estimate* made by the patient, and the patient is asked to account for the difference between the two (with the original estimate typically being much higher than the cumulative probability). You can write this analysis on a dry-erase board or flipchart, and it can also be copied onto a clipboard by the patient, so that the patient can refer to it in the future and also use it to practice the technique as other examples emerge in the weeks ahead.

Overestimations of the *severity of the consequences* of something bad happening can also be addressed using various cognitive techniques, the most common of which is to perform a *behavioral experiment*. For example, a behavioral experiment for patients who constantly rewrite e-mails before sending them or essays before turning them in may be to deliberately write an e-mail and/ or essay with typos and other errors in it and then send it/turn it in without correcting it to see whether their feared predicted consequences occur. The important thing to remember here is that the experiment should be well designed before being carried out—including being sure to operationalize the feared consequence(s) ahead of time and obtain ratings of the patient's strength of belief in them. As a consequence, you and the patient will be able to accurately assess the outcome afterward, re-rate the patient's strength of belief in them (looking for reductions), and generate alternative hypotheses that are more balanced and realistic.

Another way to address overestimations of the severity of the consequences of something bad happening is to have the patient seek information from a reliable source (e.g., an expert or a well-established website). In this case, the patient would either research the consequences or ask for the expert's opinion—being sure to focus on what would actually be expected to occur as opposed to all of the possibilities that could occur. For example, a patient who is afraid of leaving the iron plugged in may refer to the owner's manual or consult an expert electrician. However, caution must be used to prevent this technique from being turned into a ritual. A typical rule of thumb is that information seeking is acceptable once and only once, and only if the patient is unaware of the answer. Any repeated checking or further inquiry of any kind should be considered a ritual and is to be prevented.

## Cognitive Techniques to Challenge Perceptions of Inflated Personal Responsibility

In some cases, despite your best effort to correct overestimations of threat/danger by challenging the likelihood and severity of the consequences (see above), patients continue to view the risk associated with their obsession as unacceptably high and therefore refuse to engage in ritual prevention. As a result, it is important for you to not only challenge overestimations of threat/

danger and the severity of the consequences, but also to examine closely what exactly makes the consequences so severe for the patient. Often, this appears to be linked to perceptions of *inflated personal responsibility.*

As with overestimation of threat/danger, to successfully challenge perceptions of inflated personal responsibility, you must be sure to address two components of responsibility that are hypothesized to inflate the patient's sense of personal responsibility: (1) overestimations of the *amount* of responsibility (e.g., if my husband chokes to death because I did not cut his meat into small enough pieces, then it is my fault!" or "If that flickering light in my neighbor's house is a fire and their house burns down, then it is my fault!"); and (2) overestimations of the predicted *consequences* of having been responsible (e.g., "If my husband chokes and dies, I will blame myself and feel guilty for the rest of my life!" or "If my neighbor's house burns down, everybody will blame me, and I will have no friends!").

Perceptions of inflated personal responsibility can be addressed using various cognitive techniques, the most common of which is called the "pie" technique. In this case, you should first ask the patient to report the percent of responsibility she would feel if the feared consequence occurred. You should then ask the patient to brainstorm a list of all other possible factors that could play a role, even if minor, in the feared consequence. After the patient is finished brainstorming, you may also suggest any obvious factors that were omitted by the patient for consideration to be added to the list. Once the list is complete, you should draw a circle (i.e., "pie") and ask the patient to fill in pieces of the pie, which will differ in size, based on the patient's ratings of each of the individual pieces' percent contribution (i.e., relative importance). Finally, after all of the other factors have been added to the pie, the patient's own contribution is added in last. Typically, only very little of the pie is left for the patient's own personal contribution to the feared consequence. You and the patient then compare this percent to the patient's original estimate, which often serves to deflate the patient's perceived personal responsibility.

Another way to address perceptions of inflated personal responsibility is to "put the appraisal on trial" using the courtroom technique. Here patients start by trying to defend their responsibility/guilt, while "only using evidence that would be admissible in court" (i.e., no personal opinions or hearsay evidence). In so doing, patients learn to focus solely on factual proof. Patients are then often asked to play the "judge" and "rule" on arguments made by you, who should voice their original fears about being responsible/guilty. In so doing, patients often learn to assess the appraisal more objectively.

Yet another way to address perceptions of inflated personal responsibility is through the double-standard technique. This technique is employed based on finding that frequently, patients hold themselves up to a standard that is much higher/stricter than the one they use for other people. Therefore, in this technique, you should ask the patient whether he would find someone else guilty if the same feared outcome happened to the other person (e.g., a good friend or a family member) in the same situation. Does the patient think other people would judge/blame the friend or family member? In considering and comparing any differences in attitudes, patients often learn to adjust/soften their standard for themselves. If this does not appear to be happening, you might also ask the patient to consider the benefits (rarely any) and costs (typically many) to maintaining their double standard.

Finally, as was the case with challenging overestimations of the severity of the consequences of something bad happening, behavioral experiments can be used to test the consequences of inflated personal responsibility. Once again, the important thing to remember is that the experiment should be well designed before being carried out, with specific predictions made of the feared consequences ahead of time, along with the patient's ratings of strength of belief in them, so that you and the patient can accurately assess the outcome afterward and also develop more balanced, objective, and realistic alternative hypotheses. However, this method is not particularly effective for patients whose feared consequences are more distal (e.g., "I'll end up in hell" or "I'll die alone") than proximal (e.g., "If I think of my therapist getting into a car accident, he will do so before our next appointment").

## Other Cognitive Techniques

Many additional cognitive techniques for treating OCD have been created, including techniques for challenging appraisals of the overimportance of thoughts (e.g., when patients believe that having a thought means it must be important and/or engage in "thought–action fusion"—believing that having a thought can cause a behavior and/or having a thought is as bad as engaging in a behavior), the need to control thoughts, the need for certainty, and perfectionism. These techniques include psychoeducation (e.g., on the nature of intrusive thoughts, appraisals), self-monitoring (e.g., intrusive thoughts and appraisals of the thoughts), a survey, the "continuum" technique (e.g., for challenging the notion that thinking something is as bad as engaging in the behavior), the "downward arrow" technique, role playing, and thought suppression experiments (e.g., pink elephant), along with many of the techniques described previously (e.g., cost–benefit analysis, behavioral experiments). Please see Appendix A as well as the References section at the end of the book for suggestions.

# ACT TECHNIQUES

Unlike cognitive therapy approaches, the aim of ACT (described in more detail in Chapters 2 and 3) is *not* to teach patients to challenge specific cognitions. Rather, ACT seeks to teach patients how to be *flexible in the way they respond* to their inner private experiences (i.e., thoughts and emotions). In terms of OCD, patients are taught that in addition to engaging in a compulsion when they experience an obsessive thought (or feel anxious), they can choose from a number of alternative responses, more adaptive responses. Although ACT also aims to help patients identify the aspects of their lives that are meaningful to them and then commit to pursuing them despite what they may be experiencing internally (e.g., obsessive thoughts and/or anxiety), this section will focus on highlighting a few of the ACT strategies that aim to teach patients with OCD ways to develop a new relationship with their thoughts. For more references on the ACT approach in general (e.g., *Acceptance and Commitment Therapy: The Process and Practice of Mindful Change* [Hayes et al., 2012]), as well as a specific application of ACT for OCD (e.g., *ACT for OCD: Abbreviated Treatment Manual* [Twohig, 2004]), see Appendix A as well as the References section at the end of the book.

One interesting technique from the ACT approach, called *creative hopelessness,* is often used early in treatment as a way of motivating patients to consider the futility in using their compulsions to manage their unwanted thoughts and emotions and instead consider alternative approaches.

This technique involves asking patients to describe all of the strategies they have used to manage their OCD prior to starting treatment and asking them to note which strategies had worked and which had not. In so doing, you are able to highlight the fact that for most patients, the tools they have developed (e.g., rituals) only seem to have provided a temporary benefit (e.g., relief), at the cost of locking them into an increasingly greater struggle with both the obsessive thoughts and the anxiety that the obsessive thoughts generate, and to encourage patients to consider the idea of trying something new and different to manage their OCD.

ACT then builds on this by using several techniques (including many creative metaphors) to illustrate how any and all attempts by patients to regulate their inner experiences may ultimately prove to be ineffective and, even worse, how the patients' attempts to control and regulate their obsessions might actually be *exacerbating* their OCD. For example, you may decide to introduce the "man in the hole" metaphor, in which you have your patient imagine that she has fallen into a hole in the ground (representing the obsessive thoughts) and the only tool she has with her to help her try to get out is a shovel (representing the rituals she has used to try to manage her obsessive thoughts and anxiety). You then use the metaphor to explain how the patient's attempts to use her rituals to reduce or control her obsessions is the same as trying to use the shovel to dig out of the hole: not only is this strategy bound to fail, but it will also likely only make the hole larger (i.e., worsen her symptoms). Thus the patient will begin to see how her attempts to control her obsessions through rituals have ultimately made the obsessions more and more central in her life and, in so doing, have allowed the obsessions to become connected to an increasing number of situations over time. With an increased awareness of the difficulty in controlling and reducing her symptoms, the patient may then be more willing to consider alternative approaches to managing her OCD.

An additional ACT technique for OCD that focuses on illustrating the limitations of thought control involves encouraging the patient to engage in thought suppression, such as to try not to think of a wonderfully warm and fresh piece of chocolate cake. Similarly, you may introduce the "two scales" metaphor in which a first scale can be used to represent the *severity of the obsessions*, while a second scale can be used to represent the patient's *willingness* to experience obsessions. You should note that although the patient has ample evidence to suggest that the first scale is very challenging to control, the second scale is much easier to control. The patient is then encouraged to focus his efforts going forward on increasing the second (willingness) scale while at the same time disengaging from the first scale (i.e., allowing the severity of the obsessions to move up and down without trying to respond to them). You should emphasize that while increasing the second (willingness) scale may or may not have any impact on the first scale, not being willing to experience obsessions appears to have played a role in increasing them or makes them more central in the patient's life. These types of exercises are all designed to try to help patients *shift their efforts* from trying to manage uncontrollable inner experiences (i.e., obsessive thoughts or the emotions associated with them) and instead accept them while trying to manage the compulsive behaviors associated with them.

ACT for OCD also includes several techniques aimed at modifying the *function* of the obsessive thought from something that the patient perceives as threatening into something seen as just another thought. For example, you may choose to include some *defusion* exercises, such as by having the patient verbalize her obsessive thought to the tune of a popular song, by using the voice of a cartoon character or by verbalizing her obsessive thought rapidly and repeatedly until it simply sounds like gibberish. In a similar vein, you may choose to introduce the "passengers on the bus" metaphor in which unruly passengers (obsessive thoughts) attempt to take control of a bus from the driver (the patient). You should note that by allowing the passengers to take control of the bus (giving attention to the obsessive thoughts), the bus can be driven off-course and/or schedule (interference with the patient's life plans) and then emphasize that the driver can regain control of the bus if she is just willing to drive the bus (focus on desired goals/values), while allowing the passengers (obsessive thoughts) to come along for the ride (not trying to suppress them), no matter how they are acting (will vary in intensity).

Additional defusion techniques from ACT include "self as context" work (e.g., the "chessboard" metaphor), as well as "contact with the present moment" (i.e., mindfulness) techniques, such as the "leaves on a stream" (or "clouds in the sky") technique in which you would encourage the patient to imagine each of his obsessive thoughts as different tree leaves that have landed on a stream (or different clouds in the sky) and are gradually and being led downstream by the gentle current (or across the sky by the gentle breeze). Finally, you may also encourage the patient to describe his obsessions in a way that indicates they are just thoughts. For example, instead of saying to himself, "What if my wife is having an affair?" you may instruct the patient to say, "*I'm having the thought that* my wife is having an affair" or even "*My OCD is telling me that* my wife is having an affair."

## METACOGNITIVE THERAPY TECHNIQUES

As described in Chapters 2 and 3, metacognitive therapy aims to help patients become aware of their metacognitive processing so that they can learn to modify maladaptive metacognitive beliefs (i.e., reactions to their thoughts), rather than the content of anxious beliefs themselves. Therefore, as is true of ACT, in metacognitive therapy the techniques focus on helping patients *alter their relationship with their thoughts*, rather than attempting to challenge or reality test the actual thoughts. While metacognitive therapy employs several therapeutic strategies (e.g., worry and rumination postponement, behavioral experiments) to help patients see how their reactions to their thoughts rather than the thoughts themselves are the problem, this section will primarily focus on highlighting a few of the many metacognitive techniques aimed at achieving "detached mindfulness"—another of the main therapeutic strategies employed in metacognitive therapy— which creates a means of relating to thoughts in a new way (Wells, 2005). It should be emphasized, however, that much like the acceptance and mindfulness techniques found in ACT and other mindfulness-based therapies, detached mindfulness is not intended to be used by patients as a means of regulating or controlling their emotions or avoiding threat (i.e., it is not intended to be used as a coping skill). Rather, the aim is to promote metacognitive and cognitive change in beliefs. For more references on the metacognitive approach in general (e.g., *Metacognitive Therapy for Anxiety and Depression* [Wells, 2011]), as well as specific applications of metacognitive therapy for OCD (e.g., "Experimental Modification of Beliefs in Obsessive–Compulsive Disorder: A Test of the Metacognitive Model" [Fisher & Wells, 2005]), see Appendix A and the References section at the end of the book.

Although many of the detached mindfulness techniques from metacognitive therapy (e.g., suppression–countersuppression experiment, clouds image, passenger train analogy, recalcitrant child analogy, verbal loop) resemble those from ACT and other mindfulness-based approaches, several are unique to metacognitive therapy. For example, the most well-known detached mindfulness technique from metacognitive therapy, called the attention training technique (ATT), is a formal attentional procedure designed to "increase metacognitive monitoring and control processes and reduce perseverative conceptual activity" (Wells, 2005, p. 350). When introducing the ATT technique, you first inform the patient that an important factor thought to maintain her emotional problems is when her attention becomes locked onto negative thoughts and events, and then note that this can be difficult for her to control. You then have the patient practice focusing her attention outwardly onto various sounds—in your office as well as outside of your office, close by and in the distance—to help the patient learn to be more flexible in focusing her attention and awareness.

Typically, six to eight different sounds are introduced as attentional targets, ideally with the sounds emanating from different spatial locations (e.g., left, right, front, rear) in relation to the patient. The exercise itself includes three components: (1) selective attention, (2) attention switching, and (3) divided attention. Each practice session generally lasts about 15 minutes, 8 of which are devoted to selective attention, 5 to attention switching, and 2 to divided attention. In addition, you should remind the patient that as the aim of the procedure is not to suppress her thoughts, if any intrusive thoughts (or sensations) occur, she should try not to react to them but instead should refocus her attention as instructed. The patient is then instructed to practice the technique at least once per day, but not to use it as a distraction or coping strategy.

Another interesting detached mindfulness technique from metacognitive therapy, called metacognitive guidance, calls for the therapist to use a series of questions during exposure to various situations (which can be neutral or anxiety-provoking) in order to "promote meta-awareness, de-centering, and freeing of attention" (Wells, 2005, p. 346). For example, you may ask the patient to go on a walk with you outside of the office, and during the walk you may ask the patient to become aware of his thoughts and images. You may then ask the patient if he can see his thoughts and the outside world at the same time and/or challenge the patient to try to hold onto a thought while also focusing on what is happening in the world around him. The patient should be instructed to ask himself whether he lives by his thoughts or by what his eyes reveal in the moment.

You may also ask the patient to engage in a free association technique to facilitate the passive observation of the ebb and flow of internal events (e.g., obsessive thoughts) that can be triggered by verbal stimuli. This promotes the "facilitation of meta-awareness, decentering, attentional detachment, and low conceptual processing" (Wells, 2005, p. 346). Here you would inform the patient that, in a moment, you will say a series of words to her. The patient should then be instructed to allow her mind to "roam freely" in response to the words and should be told not to attempt to control or analyze anything, but rather to merely watch how her mind responds without trying to influence anything, no matter what happens. The technique usually starts with neutral or positive words (e.g., apple, birthday, seaside, tree, bicycle, summertime, and roses), with the eventual goal of having the patient apply this strategy (just watching what her mind does without getting actively caught up in any thinking process) to her obsessive thoughts.

Finally, you may employ the "tiger" technique to help the patient practice detached mindfulness to spontaneous intrusive images by observing the nonvolitional aspects of imagery. Much like the other techniques described above, this technique is typically introduced using a neutral image and then is applied to the spontaneous intrusive images that the patient experiences. You would ask the patient to conjure up an image of a tiger in his mind and then passively watch how the image develops over time while doing nothing to influence it. In other words, the patient should watch the tiger without making any attempt to influence or change the tiger's behavior (e.g., he should not try make it move or change in any way, while also allowing it to move or change on its own). You should then wait a few minutes before asking the patient about the movements the tiger made and whether he made it move.

---

## TAKE-HOME MESSAGE

Although the Ex/RP continues to be the "gold-standard" psychological treatment for patients with OCD, not all patients are motivated to try—or respond positively to—Ex/RP. As a result, you should also be careful to *customize the treatment to fit the particular needs of the patient* rather than try to *force the patient to fit the therapy*. In other words, you should begin treatment with a customized case formulation and treatment plan as well as an understanding that it is likely, at various times throughout the treatment, that the case formulation and treatment plan will need to be adjusted as new data are obtained. Logically then, you must be willing to consider adjusting the treatment goals, the pacing of the treatment, and the techniques being used, and in order to address each patient's specific needs and life circumstances.

Fortunately, in addition to Ex/RP and medications, expert consensus guidelines suggest that a number of other psychological techniques and interventions can be used to augment Ex/RP. These include several cognitive techniques, as well techniques derived from ACT and metacognitive therapy, each of which has growing empirical support in the treatment of OCD. If there is one theme unifying all of these additional approaches, it appears to be the encouragement of patients to be *flexible in the way they respond* to their inner private experiences (i.e., thoughts and emotions), such as by examining their thoughts about the thoughts (e.g., appraisals, metacognitive beliefs), by being mindful of thoughts, by detaching or "defusing" from thoughts, and by accepting their thoughts rather than reality-testing or challenging the thoughts in some way.

As such, these approaches can readily be used as *optional* components in this treatment planner, as long as you are clear about how they fit with Ex/RP (e.g., all of the strategies—in Ex/RP as well as the other approaches—aim to *teach patients how to develop a new relationship with their thoughts*). As such, these techniques may be included in any order, with or without adaptation, prior to commencing Ex/RP, while engaging the patient in Ex/RP, or after completing a course of Ex/RP. As always, the decision of whether to include these supplementary techniques, and if so, which ones to include and when to include them, will depend on your ever-evolving case conceptualization of the patient's OCD and assessment (subjective and/or objective) of how successfully the therapy is unfolding.

# CHAPTER 15

# Case Example

## PRETREATMENT

### Contact and Phone Screen

Sam, a 29-year-old, employed and married man, called to inquire about the possibility of receiving treatment for what he had "self-diagnosed" as OCD, after conducting a thorough Internet search on his symptoms and then finding my contact information online. During a brief phone screen, Sam reported that while he had always performed "little rituals" for as long as he could remember, it was not until recently that he felt they were getting out of control and starting to impair his life. He linked the exacerbation of his symptoms to two main events that had occurred earlier in the year: (1) the birth of his daughter and (2) a promotion he received at work. Sam reported that his symptoms currently included excessive checking rituals at work and at home, as well as a growing concern about germs and contamination, and other "more disturbing images and thoughts" (which he stated he would prefer to discuss in person). He rated his symptom severity currently at an 8/10, which was the worst they had been in the past year (with the best they had been being about a 4/10 in the past year).

Sam reported that he had never been in treatment of any kind for OCD or any other psychological issues and, in fact, had considered himself to be quite successful owing to his "mental toughness"—until this year. Along with self-diagnosing OCD, Sam had already read about evidence-based treatments for OCD and decided that since he did not want to take any medications, he would start with CBT. Sam appeared to have a basic understanding of what the treatment would entail, and he rated both his motivation and readiness to try CBT at 10/10, adding that he would "do everything it took to get to the appointments, complete the assignments, and get his life back on track." Sam denied any abuse of drugs or alcohol, although he stated that his alcohol use had initially increased as he attempted to "take the edge off" his symptoms but noted that he had since stopped drinking entirely. Sam denied any current suicidal or homicidal ideation. He stated that although he had told his wife about his symptoms (who was supportive), he had not told anyone else out of a fear of being judged. Given his urgency and motivation to get started, he was scheduled for an intake evaluation the same week.

## Intake Evaluation—Part I

Sam arrived on time for the intake evaluation. Upon arrival, he completed a basic demographic form, was given a Health Insurance Portability and Accountability Act (HIPAA) policy to review and an informed consent form, which he quickly read and signed after declaring that he had no questions about its contents. He was neatly dressed and well groomed, appearing his stated age. He appeared slightly anxious and fidgety, but a brief mental status examination found nothing remarkable across all domains.

Sam was then led through a general clinical evaluation, which included gathering more identifying information and detailing the course and history of his OCD. During this portion of the intake evaluation, Sam reported that he could remember engaging in some ordering and arranging rituals as a child, counting and tapping rituals as a teenager in high school, and engaging in some rereading and rewriting rituals when he was in college. Sam stressed, however, that at no time did any of these rituals cause him a great deal of distress or interfere with his life in any way. He added that he had always managed to "keep them under control" and, in fact, had excelled in high school and college, and even went on to complete an MBA at a very prestigious school of business.

Sam reported that he began to notice his OCD symptoms take a turn for the worse earlier this year, linking the exacerbation of his symptoms to the birth of his daughter and his job promotion. Sam explained that ever since his daughter was born, he had been experiencing obsessive thoughts about "something bad" happening to her, including: getting sick from germs or contaminants, falling and injuring herself, and even being attacked by strangers. This had resulted in an increase in Sam's cleaning and washing rituals (e.g., himself, his house, his wife, and his daughter), as well as checking rituals to make sure his daughter was safe (e.g., checking on her repeatedly after she was put to bed, taking her temperature, overwashing her clothes, limiting who and what she could come into contact with, washing his hands excessively before he held her).

After some gentle prodding, Sam hesitantly added that he had also been experiencing obsessive thoughts about harming his daughter himself. Sam was extremely ashamed to report these thoughts and was clearly upset by them, emphasizing that he found them horrific and repugnant and stating emphatically that he could never imagine ever wanting to harm another person—let alone his own sweet, innocent child. As a result of these obsessions, however, he was starting to avoid being left alone to care for his daughter, would insist that his wife accompany him when he checked on her after she was put to bed, and constantly sought reassurance from his wife that he was not a bad person and would not harm/had not harmed his daughter in some way. I commended Sam for mentioning these fears and normalized them before continuing on with the intake evaluation.

Finally, Sam reported that although his symptoms were initially confined to his daughter, a couple of months after his daughter was born he received a "big promotion" at work, which put him in a new role and gave him new responsibilities. It was shortly after this time that Sam began to obsess and ritualize more about his work (e.g., excessively checking over reports he had to turn in, as well as e-mails and memos he had to send out) and while at work (e.g., wiping down his desk for fear of contaminants, calling home to check on his daughter). The rituals were growing more frequent and intense over time to the point that they were now causing him a significant amount of distress as well as interfering with his ability to function at work (e.g., he was starting to miss deadlines for projects, was not responding to e-mails, and had been keeping his office door closed in order to discourage people from entering it and contaminating it).

Sam denied ever having received psychiatric treatment, reported a clean medical history (e.g., he recently had had a physical, with no significant findings, was not taking any medications, had no history of major illnesses or injuries), and said that he had been into "clean living" for most of his life (e.g., he always maintained a healthy diet, exercised regularly, and had never used any recreational drugs). Sam did report that he drank alcohol socially, observing that it had "almost become a problem" a couple of months ago, when he began to increase his drinking (at night) in an attempt to "take the edge off" his anxiety and "quiet down" his thoughts. He added, however, that this behavior only lasted a few days before he realized it was a bad strategy and so he stopped drinking entirely because he wanted to get his life in check before he would consider drinking again.

Regarding his family psychiatric and medical history, Sam noted that while he was unaware of anyone in the family ever having been treated for a psychological disorder, both of his parents were anxious and, looking back, he could see how each had at least some traits of OCD. Sam reported that he also had one sister who had suffered from depression after the birth of her first child, but added that she had received treatment for it and was now doing well. Other than that, he could not recall any psychiatric or medical history in his family.

In terms of his personal and social history, Sam reported that he had been born and raised in the area and had lived in the same house until he left for college at age 18. He denied experiencing any significant negative events during his early years, emphasizing that he felt loved and supported by his parents, who always wanted the best for him. He added that he did well in high school and college, making friends easily and graduating with high honors before completing an MBA at a very prestigious college a few years ago. After graduating with his MBA, Sam landed his current job in finance, which he was very much enjoying (and excelling at) until his OCD symptoms flared up a few months ago. Sam also reported that he had been happily married to his wife for the past five years, adding that they had met and fallen in love in their first year of college and not been apart ever since that time. Sam reported that his wife was aware of his symptoms, was very supportive of him, and was behind him 100% in terms of his seeking help. Sam also reported that he had a large group of friends—both at work and outside of work but stated that he was not comfortable telling any of them about his symptoms. He admitted, however, that a few of his close male friends had spotted him performing rituals from time to time and teased him about them. Sam denied having any legal history (no charges or arrests).

As it was nearing the end of the session, Sam was given a preliminary DSM diagnosis of OCD, with good insight (300.3[F42]) and was assigned a comprehensive, empirically based self-report measures packet to complete for homework.

## Intake Evaluation—Part II

Sam returned the next week reporting feeling good about having started the process of getting help, but adding that nothing had changed in terms of his OCD symptom severity. He had completed the homework (a comprehensive, empirically based self-report measures packet), did not have any questions about the previous visit, and had no significant events to report since the last session—

although he did note that since having the discussion with me about his harm obsessions, he had been trying not to avoid being around his daughter, even though it was causing him great distress.

I then completed the Mini-International Neuropsychiatric Interview (a short, structured diagnostic interview) with Sam to confirm the diagnosis of OCD (he did meet the criteria) and assess for the presence of any comorbid conditions (none were found). I then administered the Y-BOCS, which not only affirmed the presence of many of the symptoms Sam had reported the previous session (e.g., aggressive obsessions, contamination obsessions, cleaning/washing compulsions, checking compulsions) but also revealed some additional symptoms that Sam had not previously considered to be part of his OCD (e.g., obsessions about symmetry and exactness, counting compulsions, and several miscellaneous obsessions and compulsions such as the need to know and remember, some superstitious fears, and having lucky numbers, excessive list-making, superstitious behaviors). His total score on the Y-BOCs was 25 (severe).

As it was nearing the end of the session, I asked Sam for feedback about the treatment process thus far, and Sam reported that he felt very good about how things had started. In particular, he appreciated the comprehensiveness of the evaluation, adding that it was nice to know that he was not crazy and that he was hopeful that he would be able to get his life back on track soon. I suggested that for homework Sam purchase a copy of *Stop Obsessing!: How to Overcome Your Obsessions and Compulsions* by Edna Foa and Reid Wilson before the next session.

Between sessions, I scored the self-report packet that Sam had completed and recorded Sam's scores on a summary page in the chart. All self-report measure scores fell in the normal range, except for his score on the OCI-R, which was a 35, approximately one-half standard deviation above the mean for patients with OCD ($\overline{X} = 28.0$; $SD = 13.53$).

## TREATMENT SESSION 1

At this and in all subsequent sessions, I began by setting a collaborative agenda with Sam. This session's agenda included:

- Check on symptoms—subjective ratings
- Administer the OCI-R
- Review homework
- Feedback on the self-report assessments
- Psychoeducation on diagnosis and prognosis and preliminary case formulation
- Psychoeducation on evidence-based treatment options
- Presentation of the CBT principles and overview of the CBT model
- Mini-motivation enhancement and commitment to the treatment
- Goals and expectations for therapy
- Questions and answers
- Homework: Rationale and assignment
- Rapport and alliance building: Feedback, summary, and a take-home message

As this was the start of the treatment sessions and Sam had never been in CBT (or any other therapy) before, I first explained the concept of collaborative agenda setting to Sam, which he understood and appreciated from his business background. The agenda (see above) was then set, after which I began by obtaining three ratings (using 0–10 scales) from Sam about his OCD since the last session: (1) how severe the OCD symptoms had been (8/10), (2) the amount of effort he had made to manage the OCD symptoms (10/10), and (3) the level of success he had had in managing the OCD symptoms (5/10). While I recorded these in the chart, I had Sam complete an evidence-based self-report measure (the OCI-R), which I then quickly scored (36), gave feedback to Sam about the score, and then noted that from now on I would leave a copy of the measure in the waiting room for Sam to complete when he arrived each week.

Next, I checked to see if Sam had completed the homework (if he had purchased a copy of *Stop Obsessing!: How to Overcome Your Obsessions and Compulsions*), which he had done—and he had even started reading the first chapter. I praised Sam for completing the homework and asked him if he had any questions about what he had read (he did not) and for a brief summary of the chapter (which Sam was able to give).

I then gave Sam feedback on the self-report package he had completed, as well as the entire assessment and evaluation phase of treatment. The feedback included psychoeducation on his diagnosis (reviewing the DSM diagnostic criteria to explain how the diagnosis was made), evidence-based treatment options (reviewing expert consensus guidelines which suggest CBT and/ or medications be considered as the first-line treatment for OCD), and a preliminary prognosis (good). Sam reiterated that he was not interested in starting a medication. I then proceeded to present an initial case formulation to Sam, including the suspected origins of his symptoms (e.g., a combination of a biological vulnerability and psychological vulnerability from his parents), a summary of the course of the disorder, a review of his current symptoms, situational factors that appear to have worsened Sam's symptoms (the birth of his daughter and his promotion at work), and a description of the main psychopathological mechanisms (e.g., maladaptive beliefs, intolerance of uncertainty, increased anxiety and stress, avoidance) that I believed were now maintaining them.

Because Sam was new to therapy, I then provided him with a written description of the principles of CBT, as well as a handout that contained both an overview of the CBT model and an explanation of how CBT would address the psychopathological mechanisms I had just described and I asked him to review them for homework.

Even though Sam appeared to be highly motivated for treatment, I next chose to conduct a mini-motivational enhancement exercise by engaging Sam in a discussion of the costs and benefits of continuing to manage the OCD in the same way he had been trying prior to entering treatment versus the costs and benefits of learning to manage the OCD in a new way through treatment. I recorded Sam's responses on a decisional balance worksheet and then made a copy of the form for Sam to review for homework. After completing this exercise, Sam appeared firmly committed to giving the treatment a try.

As it was nearing the end of the session, I asked Sam to describe his goals for treatment and expectations for me, and worked with him to ensure that his goals and expectations were specific and realistic. Sam ended up with three main goals for treatment: (1) eliminate the need to perform rituals, (2) increase his ability to tolerate obsessions, and (3) reduce the severity of his OCD by half (e.g., OCI-R score of 18 or less and Y-BOCS of 13 or less).

I then asked Sam if he had any questions (he did not), before reviewing the rationale and importance of homework compliance on treatment outcome, and collaborating with Sam on the homework, which included continuing to read *Stop Obsessing!*, reviewing the psychoeducational handouts, reviewing the decisional balance worksheet, and beginning to monitor his OCD symptoms using a symptom monitoring form (which I reviewed with him).

Finally, I continued to build rapport and alliance by asking Sam for feedback about the process so far ("We're right on track, and I am excited to get started with the treatment"), along with both a summary and a take-home message from the session.

## TREATMENT SESSION 2

Treatment Session 2's agenda included:

- Completion of the OCI-R
- Check on symptoms—subjective ratings
- Review of the homework
- Review of the CBT model
- Modification of the general CBT model to explain OCD
- Rationale for CBT for OCD
- Brief overview of the treatment
- Questions and answers
- Homework
- Rapport and alliance building: Feedback, summary, and take-home message

Sam arrived on time and completed the OCI-R, which I had left waiting for him in the waiting room. After collaboratively setting the agenda, I quickly scored this measure and gave Sam feedback about the score (35, a reduction of 1 point from the previous session).

Then, as was the case at the start of the previous session, I asked Sam to provide the same three ratings (using 0–10 scales) about his OCD since the last session: (1) how severe the OCD symptoms had been (8/10), (2) the amount of effort he had made to manage the OCD symptoms (9/10), and (3) the level of success he had had in managing the OCD symptoms (4/10). I recorded these ratings in the chart, noting that Sam had slipped slightly in his effort (Sam responded that he had been extra busy at work, which had negatively impacted his resolve to fight his OCD at times) and, perhaps as a result, had also slipped slightly in his reported success in managing the OCD. Sam agreed with the observation and indicated that he would work to increase his effort in the following week.

Next, I checked on the homework, first reviewing Sam's progress on the self-help book (*Stop Obsessing!*), which Sam had continued to read, did not have any questions about, and was able to summarize well. I then asked if Sam had reviewed the psychoeducational handouts (he had, did not have any questions about them, and was able to give me a good summary of them) and the Decisional Balance Worksheet (he had, and had even added some other items with help from his wife). Finally, I checked on whether Sam had monitored his OCD symptoms on the symptom monitoring form (he had). I spent some time reviewing this form, looking for new triggers, and assessing where Sam had slipped the most.

I then reviewed the general CBT model with Sam (using Socratic questioning), making sure Sam understood the difference between thoughts, feelings, and actions, along with the bidirectional connection between each one of these modalities to the other two. Once it was clear that Sam understood the general CBT model, I (using a dry-erase board) then modified it into a CBT model of his OCD, defining each of the components and emphasizing the role that his rituals played in reducing his anxiety in the short-term while also increasing the salience of the triggers and thoughts that were ultimately perpetuating his anxiety in the long term.

I then presented a detailed rationale for using a cognitive-behavioral approach for treating Sam's OCD and showed Sam how, by learning to test his predictions and tolerate his anxiety *without engaging in rituals*, he could "break the cycle" of his OCD and begin to get his life back on track. Sam reported that he was excited to learn how his OCD appeared to have been maintained over time, while also being slightly nervous about starting treatment.

I then provided Sam with a brief overview of the treatment plan, in part to address his nervousness; in part to demonstrate that while we would be following a structured, evidence-based plan, it would be customized to Sam's unique history and symptoms; and in part to show him that I anticipated a time when the treatment would end as our goals would have been reached.

I then addressed several questions that Sam had about the structure and pace of the treatment before collaborating with him on the homework for the week, which included continuing to read the self-help book, continuing to monitor his OCD symptoms on the symptom monitoring form, and reviewing his notes on the CBT model of OCD.

Finally, I continued to build our rapport and alliance by asking Sam for feedback on the session, as well as a summary and a take-home message from it.

## TREATMENT SESSION 3

Treatment Session 3's agenda included:

- Completion of the OCI-R
- Check on symptoms—subjective ratings
- Review of the homework
- Review of the CBT model of OCD and rationale for CBT for OCD
- Explanation of the concept of SUDS and creation of a personalized scale
- Generation of items for the exposure hierarchy
- Homework
- Rapport and alliance building: Feedback, summary, and a take-home message

Sam arrived on time and once again completed the OCI-R, which I quickly scored (35, showing no change from the previous session) and then gave him feedback.

I then asked Sam for the three ratings on his OCD since the last session, which he reported as follows: (1) severity of his OCD symptoms (9/10), (2) amount of effort he had made to manage his OCD symptoms (10/10), and (3) level of success he had had in managing his OCD symptoms (3/10). I recorded these scores in the chart, observing that while Sam had increased his effort this week, his perceived success in managing the OCD had dropped another point and, perhaps relatedly, his rating of the overall severity had increased by a point. Sam agreed with the observation, noting that although he really tried hard to fight the OCD this week, it had "gotten the better of [him]" and appeared to him to be worsening (owing to the fact that he could not manage the symptoms as well because he seemed to experience more obsessions and the rituals he felt compelled to complete had taken up more of his time). I normalized this experience and reinforced Sam for his efforts. We also looked for any factors that may have influenced his symptoms (but could not find anything out of the norm).

I then checked on the homework, first reviewing Sam's progress on the self-help book (*Stop Obsessing!*), which he had continued to read and demonstrated a good understanding of the content. I then asked if he had reviewed his notes on the CBT model for OCD (he had). Finally, I checked whether Sam had continued to monitor his OCD symptoms on the symptom monitoring form (he had). I spent some time reviewing this form with him, looking for new triggers and noting where he had seemed to have the most difficulty managing his OCD in the past week.

I then asked Sam to walk me through the CBT model of his OCD, as well as the rationale for using CBT to treat OCD, by engaging him in a brief role play in which I took on the role of a patient and Sam took on the role of the therapist. He was able to present the model and rationale quite well, and I needed to add only minor additions/corrections after the role play was ended.

Next, I introduced the rationale for creating a SUDS for Sam and then personalized the scale for him by having him generate anchors for the 0/10 (relaxing on a beach), 5/10 (important meeting at work), and 10/10 (wife about to give birth) levels on the scale. Once the SUDS was complete, I worked with Sam to generate items for the exposure hierarchy, using information gathered from the intake evaluation (e.g., the Y-BOCS checklist). Together, we were able to come up with approximately 15 items of varying SUDS levels that we agreed would be used for the Ex/RP portion of the treatment.

As the session time was winding down, I spent the remaining time first addressing questions that Sam had about the Ex/RP phase of the treatment and then collaborating with Sam on setting the homework for the week (e.g., continuing to read the self-help book, continuing to monitor his OCD symptoms using the symptom monitoring form, reviewing the CBT model for OCD and rationale for Ex/RP, and examining the hierarchy). Finally, I continued to strengthen our rapport and alliance by asking Sam for feedback on the session, as well as a summary and a take-home message from it.

## TREATMENT SESSION 4

Treatment Session 4's agenda included:

- Completion of the OCI-R
- Check on symptoms—subjective ratings
- Review of the homework
- Quick review of the CBT model of OCD and rationale for Ex/RP
- Review of the concept of SUDS and SUDS ratings
- Review and finalization of the exposure hierarchy
- Motivational enhancement (added after check on symptoms—see below)
- Preparation for Ex/RP
- Outline of session structure for Ex/RP

- Introduction of ritual prevention between sessions
- Homework
- Rapport and alliance building: Feedback, summary, and a take-home message

Sam once again arrived on time and completed the OCI-R, scoring a 37 (two points higher than the previous session). Sam explained that all of the recent focus on his symptoms, combined with having to create a hierarchy for Ex/RP last week, seemed to have intensified his symptoms. This was confirmed when I asked Sam for his three ratings on his OCD since the last session, which he reported as follows: (1) severity of the OCD symptoms: (10/10), (2) effort made to manage the OCD symptoms (7/10), and (3) success in managing the OCD symptoms (2/10).

I recorded these scores in the chart next to the previous scores, validating Sam's reaction as common once patients begin to focus on their OCD and embrace the idea that they will soon be facing their fears. When I asked about the decrease in effort made and success in managing the symptoms, Sam reported that at times he was "too tired to fight it." As it seemed to be "much more powerful" this week, he "just gave in" and ritualized. I also normalized these thoughts and suggested that we revisit Sam's decisional balance during the session to see if we could increase his level of motivation and commitment to the treatment, before starting Ex/RP.

I then checked on the homework, first reviewing Sam's progress on the self-help book (*Stop Obsessing!*), which Sam reported he had *not* read this week, first citing he was "too busy," then adding that he was "too overwhelmed" by his symptoms, and finally admitting that he had lost motivation to read about OCD, given how intense his OCD symptoms were this week. I validated his reaction and then collaborated with Sam to problem-solve some alternative ways (cognitively and behaviorally) in which he might approach this portion of the homework in the future, in the event he was to feel the same way again. We also agreed that Sam should plan a specific day and time to reinitiate the reading and set a more manageable target for the amount of reading he would do on the first night this week (e.g., spend 15 minutes skimming the last five pages he read last week to refresh his memory before moving on to new material).

Sam also had not completed any self-monitoring of his OCD symptoms on the symptom monitoring form, so I collaborated with him to problem-solve some alternative ways (cognitively and behaviorally) in which he might also approach this portion of the homework in the future, if he was to feel the same way again. Given that Sam had also reported that this was a particularly challenging week (and to get him refocused on completing the Self-Monitoring Form), I decided to review several instances in which Sam struggled and had Sam practice entering these on the Self-Monitoring Form as each one was reviewed.

Not surprisingly, Sam also reported that he had not reviewed the CBT model for OCD or the rationale for Ex/RP. I therefore had him describe each in session to ensure his understanding of them (he did this thoroughly and with only minimal correction). Sam had managed to review the SUDS and hierarchy created in the last session and was able to describe the rationale behind creating the scale and using it to guide the hierarchy construction as well as Ex/RP. Sam also reported that he had no items to add to the hierarchy, adding that it was making him anxious to think about facing each of the items in such a short time—especially those items near the top of the hierarchy. Once again I normalized this response, while also asking Sam to describe what he was predicting would happen, so that these predictions could be examined and tested at a later date.

I then presented Sam with a copy of the hierarchy, which I had arranged in order from highest to lowest SUDS rating, and I asked him to review and approve the final arrangement of items. After seeing the items arranged in order, Sam decided to make a couple of minor modifications (increases) to the SUDS ratings on two items, which I immediately edited, and I then reprinted the final version for Sam and for the chart.

Since I had already performed a quick review of the CBT model of OCD and rationale for Ex/RP, as well as a review of the concept of SUDS and creating the SUDS scale while doing the homework review, this part of the agenda was considered complete and we moved on to the item added (revisiting of Sam's decisional balance) during the check on his symptoms at the beginning of the session. Taking out a copy of the Decisional Balance Worksheet Sam completed with me during the "mini-motivation enhancement and commitment to the treatment" section of treatment Session 1, we reviewed the responses Sam had given, connecting his struggles during the previous week to the short-term costs of learning to manage the OCD in a new way through treatment while also reviewing the long-term costs of continuing to manage the OCD in the same way, along with the long-term benefits of learning to manage the OCD in a new way through treatment. Sam found this review very helpful and was able to recommit to the treatment. He stated that he would keep a copy of the Decisional Balance Worksheet accessible and would review it between sessions and whenever he found himself wavering in his motivation and/or commitment or struggling to complete an assignment.

I then began to prepare Sam for the Ex/RP phase of the treatment, which would commence at the next visit. This included informing him of how the Ex/RP sessions would be structured (e.g., quick check-in on symptoms and homework, with the bulk of the visit for Ex/RP practice) and what would be expected of him, both during the session and between the sessions. I then collaborated with Sam to select the item that would be used for the initial Ex/RP session, ultimately selecting an item with a SUDS value of 4 (writing and sending out an interoffice memo electronically without doing a spell/grammar check).

Given how Sam had responded between sessions after creating the hierarchy, I decided to engage him in a brief discussion of how he might notice more feelings of anxiety between sessions as the first Ex/RP session date approached, and connected it to the CBT model. I also framed it as a positive sign of change, and I reminded him to review the Decisional Balance Worksheet, if necessary. I also instructed Sam to not make any special advance "arrangements" (i.e., engage in "preventative" rituals before the Ex/RP session, such as crafting out his memo ahead of time) to counter his feared consequences of the upcoming exposure task.

I then provided Sam with the rationale for striving for 100% ritual prevention between sessions from this point on, via a review of the CBT model of OCD, with an emphasis on the important role that rituals had played in maintaining his OCD. I then acknowledged that while initially anxiety-provoking, Sam's ritual prevention efforts would provide several benefits in the long term (which I reviewed with him). Then I collaborated with Sam to generate specific examples of how he would strive to prevent his particular rituals at home and in the office, and I turned these into a "rules for ritual prevention" form for him to review whenever necessary.

I noted that while slips would likely happen along the way from this point on. Sam should always be striving for a 100% effort at resisting his urges to ritualize. I addressed his questions and concerns, which included what to do in the event of a slip (e.g., view as challenges, record on the Self-Monitoring Form, and proceed to "undo" the slip by re-exposing himself immediately to the situation or thought that generated the ritual), and how to tell a ritual from a "normal" concern (e.g., what is an appropriate concern for a new parent and person in a new role at work?). For the latter, rather than make specific rules, I suggested Sam ask himself whether whatever he was about to do would help him reach his treatment goals.

As the session was coming to an end, I spent the remaining time collaborating with Sam on setting the homework for the week (e.g., reading of the self-help book, striving for 100% ritual prevention, recording any slips on the symptom monitoring form, review the Decisional Balance Worksheet and rules for ritual prevention form) as well as continuing to strengthen our rapport and therapeutic alliance by asking him for a summary and take-home message from the session, along with feedback on the session and my performance as his therapist.

## TREATMENT SESSIONS 5–14: TEN SESSIONS OF EX/RP

The agenda for treatment Sessions 5–14 followed roughly the same structure:

- Completion of the OCI-R
- Check on symptoms—OCD severity, effort and success at 100% ritual prevention
- Review of the homework
- In-session Ex/RP
- Motivational enhancement (if necessary)
- New homework
- Rapport and alliance maintenance: Feedback, summary, and a take-home message

In addition, the agenda for Session 14 included a review of the rationale for the home visit along with preparation for it.

For Sam, addressing his slip in motivation during Session 4 proved very helpful, as he returned to Session 5 (and all subsequent sessions) with a high motivation and commitment to do the work necessary to create change in his life. He consistently arrived on time, completing the OCI-R before the start of each session, which I would record and graph for him. After a brief uptick in his OCI-R score at the start of Ex/RP in Session 5, Sam was pleased to see his scores begin to fall at the start of Session 6, as well as with nearly every subsequent session.

Parallel with this progress, Sam noticed that his self-reported ratings of his OCD severity began to decrease with each additional Ex/RP session. He was pleasantly surprised to find that he could honestly report that he was needing to put less and less effort into ritual prevention, while still being able to achieve nearly 100% ritual prevention (he continued to experience the occasional slip at home and at work). Sam also found it helpful and motivating to see my graphs of these scores, as it allowed him to see the gains he was making and incentivized him to continue to build on these gains each week.

Sam was exceptional in his dedication to engage in Ex/RP within each session, collaborating with me on generating each week's representative item and gradually taking the lead in running the Ex/RP portion of the session on his own (i.e., even without my needing to role-model for him). Sam was also extremely compliant with the between-session (homework) Ex/RP assignments (a review of his Ex/RP Practice Records each week showed he was practicing for at least an hour each day, either at home, at work, or both at home and work) and would often return with insights and ideas to share with me on how to maximize his gains. He also finished reading the self-help book, which he thought was an excellent supplement for the ideas and concepts covered in the treatment, and he was diligent about recording any slips in his ritual prevention, as well as problem-solving ways in which he would prevent a similar slip from occurring. For Sam, adhering to this structure and plan, with only the occasional reminder from me to review his Decisional Balance Worksheet, the CBT model for OCD, and the rationale for treatment (all for maintaining motivation and commitment), was sufficient to help him achieve all three of his treatment goals.

As mentioned above, by the time Sam reached Session 14, he was feeling very confident in his ability to manage the OCD and could see the end in sight for his treatment. As such, I suggested that the next session be a home visit, so that I could observe Sam practicing Ex/RP with his daughter present and also do an assessment for any potential remaining triggers or commonly avoided situations in the home. As Sam agreed with this suggestion, some time was saved at the end of Session 14 to prepare for the home visit. This included setting a rough agenda for the visit in advance, rules and expectations for the home visit, how to ensure, and who else should be present (along with his daughter, the patient was excited to have his wife present, so she could see how far he'd come).

## TREATMENT SESSION 15: HOME VISIT

Treatment Session 15's agenda included:

- Brief reminder of the session agenda and structure
- Completion of the OCI-R
- Brief check on symptoms—OCD severity, effort and success at 100% ritual prevention
- Brief review of the homework
- In-home assessment of triggers and/or avoidances
- Brief check on the patient's motivation to engage in Ex/RP
- In-home Ex/RP
- Final homework
- Rapport and alliance building: Feedback, summary, and a take-home message
- Preparing for the final session (relapse prevention)

As had become the norm with the in-office visits, Sam was prepared and eager for my arrival for the home visit. After a brief review of the structure and agenda, I had Sam complete the OCI-R, before having him report on the severity of his OCD since the last session, as well as his effort and success at 100% ritual prevention. I recorded these scores in the chart next to the previous scores, and I noted that I would graph his results at the start of the final session.

I then did a brief check on the homework, first reviewing Sam's few slips on the symptom monitoring form and then reviewing how he addressed the slips in order to undo them as well as prevent them from recurring in the future, and finally reviewing Sam's Ex/RP Practice Records for the week.

Next, I had Sam (with his wife present) do a walkthrough of the home, asking him (and his wife) to indicate objects, areas, and situations that had been triggers for his OCD symptoms. I had Sam give each item they encountered two SUDS ratings (past and current) and occasionally had Sam demonstrate how he had confronted the trigger during his at-home Ex/RP. I also asked him to note any objects, areas, and situations that could become triggers in the future. Finally, given that Sam had been concerned with contamination, I asked if he had a "safe zone" in the home (in this case, he had initially had two such areas—his bed and his daughter's room—but had already worked on contaminating them as part of his at-home assignment work).

I then conducted a brief check on Sam's motivation to engage in the final, at-home Ex/RP assignment, which involved feeding his daughter, giving her a bath, and putting her to bed (an item that was at the top of his hierarchy that he had been unable to complete on his own at home). Although Sam still rated his anxiety as moderately high (6/10) for this item, he was motivated to try this "once and for all" as it was the "last obstacle" in the way of his success. He predicted that his SUDS would "likely hit 100" during the Ex/RP, and while he initially denied he had any other feared predictions, he quickly corrected himself, admitted that he was worried that in caring for her, he would harm her in some way (e.g., he could burn her mouth during the bottle feeding or even worse, he could burn her and/or drown her during the bath or suffocate her after putting her to bed). He rated his strength in these beliefs as 3/10, 5/10, and 5/10, respectively, noting, however, that this was in part because I and his wife were present and were monitoring the situation. Sam reported that his typical coping strategy had been to avoid taking on these tasks, but since he would not be able to avoid them this time, he would likely be overly cautious about testing the temperature of the formula in the bottle and the water in the bath, as well as wanting to leave the bathroom and bedroom doors open so that his wife and I could monitor him during those portions of the Ex/RP. Sam reported, however, a high (10/10) willingness to prevent the use of these coping strategies, rituals, and safety behaviors.

Sam was instructed to begin the Ex/RP with his daughter, and to test out his predictions, he agreed to do the exercise without me or his wife present (we waited in another area of the house). Sam completed the exercise and returned to the room where I and his wife were waiting, and proudly reported a postexposure SUDS rating of 1/10. Further questioning indicated that Sam's maximum SUDS actually briefly reached a 9/10 on two occasions: when he was alone with his daughter in the bathroom and again when he was alone with her in the bedroom. In each of these situations, however, Sam's SUDS dropped fairly quickly, as he learned he could experience his obsessive thoughts and not act on them. As a result, he noted that all of his feared predictions did not happen, and re-rated his strength in these beliefs as 1/10, 3/10, and 3/10, respectively. Sam was also able to come up with more rational alternative beliefs for each scenario, reported only a mild urge to ritualize (i.e., check on his daughter; 3/10), with a high willingness (10/10) to prevent himself from checking on her.

As the home visit was coming to an end, I spent the remaining time collaborating with Sam on setting the final homework assignments. These included continuing to strive for 100% ritual prevention and recording any slips on the monitoring form, along with a description of how he undid them and a plan to prevent them from happening again in the future; repeating the in-home *in vivo* Ex/RP, only this time without his wife at home; and completing a set of end-of-treatment questionnaires (which I gave to him). As usual, I also asked Sam for a summary and a take-home message from the session, along with feedback on how he felt the session went and how I performed in my role as his therapist.

## TREATMENT SESSION 16: RELAPSE PREVENTION AND TERMINATION

Treatment Session 16's agenda included:

- Final completion of the OCI-R
- Final check on symptoms—OCD severity, effort and success at 100% ritual prevention
- Readministration of the Y-BOCS
- Final review of the homework
- Final ratings of original exposure hierarchy
- Discussion of relapse prevention
- Ongoing homework
- Rapport and alliance building: Feedback, summary, and a take-home message
- Plan "booster" session

Sam arrived on time for the final session and completed the OCI-R. I quickly scored it (13) at the start of the session, entered it into the chart, and produced a summary graph for Sam to keep as a reminder of the progress he made in the treatment. I also noted how this score meant that Sam had achieved one of his treatment goals (an OCI-R score of 18 or less) he had set at the end of treatment Session 1.

Next, I asked Sam to give a final report on the severity of his OCD (2/10), as well as his effort at 100% ritual prevention (2/10—which he explained was good, as it took less effort to keep himself from ritualizing now) and success at ritual prevention (10/10). I recorded these scores in the chart next to the previous scores, and I also produced a summary graph of these results for Sam to keep as a reminder of the progress he made in the treatment. In addition, I noted how Sam had achieved another of the goals he had set at the end of treatment Session 1 (eliminate the need to perform rituals).

I then readministered the Y-BOCS with Sam, doing a quick review of the checklist in its entirety while paying particular attention to each of the obsessions and compulsions he had endorsed at the start of treatment. This affirmed the progress he had made in treatment by demonstrating how many of the symptoms Sam had originally endorsed were no longer present and by the total score now being 11 (mild). Once again, I noted how Sam had achieved the third of his three goals set at the end of treatment Session 1 (Y-BOCS of 13 or less).

The next item on the agenda involved conducting a final check on the homework. Sam was proud to report that he had made it through the entire week being 100% successful at ritual prevention for the first time. As such, he did not have any entries to review on the monitoring form. Sam added that he was especially proud because he accomplished this with less effort than he had previously put into fighting the rituals, and because he accomplished this feat while repeating the in-home *in vivo* Ex/RP exercise several times, without his wife present. Even more impressive was the fact that after reviewing Sam's Ex/RP Practice Records, it was evident that feeding and bathing his daughter, as well as putting her to bed on his own, were no longer making him as anxious. I praised him for his efforts while reviewing what he had learned from the exercises. Finally, I collected the set of end-of-treatment questionnaires that I had given to Sam at the end of the home visit (and Sam had completed between sessions). I noted that I would score them and would give Sam a summary of how his scores had changed on the measures between the start and end of treatment.

I then reviewed the original exposure hierarchy with Sam, asking him to make final SUDS ratings on each of the items. Once this was complete, I entered the items into the chart and produced a copy for Sam as a reminder of the progress he had made in treatment and as a tool to be used to aid him in his future relapse prevention efforts.

The bulk of the remainder of the session focused on relapse prevention and included a final review of the CBT model of OCD and the rationale for treatment; a lesson on how to differentiate a lapse from a relapse; a discussion on the importance of continuing to use the skills learned in treatment; identification of upcoming high-risk situations; planning on how to fill in the time freed up in Sam's day owing to the decrease in his symptoms; and a discussion of how to taper off ritual prevention and ease back into "normal" behavior.

This led naturally into a discussion of ongoing homework, which included regularly reviewing all of the notes and handouts from the treatment sessions as well as the self-help book; beginning the tapering of ritual prevention and return to "normal" behavior; continuing Ex/RP for all items on the hierarchy that still generated more than mild (3/10+) anxiety; finding naturalistic opportunities to engage in Ex/RP; noting any slips on the Self-Monitoring Form along with an explanation of how he undid them and how he would prevent a similar slip in the future; creating a plan for any high-risk situations coming up; and beginning to fill in the time freed up by the decrease in symptoms with activities he valued (e.g., time with his daughter and wife).

As the session was nearly over, I spent the remaining time asking Sam for feedback on the entire treatment process, as well as a final summary and a take-home message from the treatment. Finally, I offered him a "booster" session to be held in one month's time in order to be able to (1) give Sam feedback on the final questionnaire packet in person, (2) keep Sam accountable for working on his OCD, (3) make sure the gains made in treatment were being maintained, and (4) problem-solve any slips/lapses. Sam was relieved and pleased to know this was an option, and he readily agreed to return in a month, assuring me he'd only have good news to report.

## TREATMENT SESSION 17: BOOSTER SESSION

Treatment Session 17's agenda included:

- Completion of the OCI-R
- Check on symptoms—OCD severity, effort and success at 100% ritual prevention
- Review of the homework
- Review of end-of-treatment self-report measures
- Ongoing relapse prevention planning
- Ongoing homework and motivation check
- Feedback, summary, and a take-home message

Sam was true to his word, returning for his booster session a month later. He arrived on time and completed the OCI-R, which I quickly scored (10) and entered into the chart. I then printed another summary graph for him to keep as a reminder of the progress he had made—in both the treatment and in the month since it ended. Next, I asked Sam to give a rating of the severity of his OCD (1/10), as well as his effort at 100% ritual prevention (1/10—again, he explained this as a good sign, as it now took much less effort for him to keep himself from ritualizing) and success at ritual prevention (10/10). I recorded these scores in the chart next to the previous scores and also produced a summary graph of these results for Sam to keep as a reminder of the progress he had made in the treatment and in the month since it ended.

Next, I provided Sam with a summary of how his scores had changed on the self-report measures he completed between the start and end of treatment (which I had scored between our meetings). As was the case with the start-of-treatment questionnaire packet, all self-report measure scores had fallen in the nonclinical range. However, this time this also included his score on the OCI-R, which had fallen to a 15, approximately one standard deviation below the mean for patients with OCD ($\overline{X} = 28.0$; $SD = 13.53$).

We then reviewed how Sam had been doing in keeping up with the homework, which included regularly reviewing all of the notes and handouts from the treatment sessions as well as the self-help book; beginning the tapering of ritual prevention and return to "normal" behavior; continuing Ex/RP for all items on the hierarchy that still generated more than mild anxiety; finding naturalistic opportunities to engage in Ex/RP; noting any slips on the Self-Monitoring Form, along with an explanation of how he undid them and how he would prevent a similar slip in the future; creating a plan for any high-risk situations coming up; and beginning to fill in the time freed up by the decrease in symptoms with activities he valued. Sam acknowledged that although he was "not perfect" when it came to the homework (e.g., he did not review the notes or book), he jokingly thought that might be a good sign (could be flexible) and emphasized that he instead had focused on "acting normal again" and not letting his OCD push him around anymore when it came to his work, family life, and daily routines. As such, he reported that he was continuing to "lean in" to situations that had previously made him anxious (e.g., bathing and changing his daughter on his own) and was proud to report that not only had he not experienced any lapses, but he had also taken advantage of several naturalistic opportunities to engage in Ex/RP that had emerged (e.g., giving his wife a night out with her friends by babysitting his daughter, sending out important documents at work without excessive checking beforehand).

The bulk of the remainder of the session focused on ongoing relapse prevention planning, including a review of the CBT model of OCD and the rationale for Ex/RP, identifying and planning how to address upcoming high-risk situations (e.g., an end-of-year report due for work, his daughter entering daycare), a review on how to differentiate a lapse from a relapse, and a reminder of the importance of continuing to use all of the skills learned in treatment. Sam was then asked to self-assign his homework, which he decided should include a more formal recurring review of his notes and handouts from the treatment, while continuing to focus his efforts on engaging in Ex/RP for any trigger (from his hierarchy or new) that generates more than mild (3/10) anxiety. I then asked Sam to rate his motivation level to continue implementing the treatment principles going forward, which he rated 10/10. I suggested that if his motivation wavered, he should review his Decisional Balance Worksheet.

As the session was nearly over, I spent the remaining time obtaining feedback on the session, as well as a summary and a take-home message. Finally, I stated that I would be closing Sam's chart after this visit, but that he was welcome to contact me again in the future if he believed he was lapsing and was struggling to come up with a plan on how to prevent a full relapse. Although Sam was relieved and pleased to know this was an option, he said that he felt confident in his ability to manage the symptoms on his own going forward and that he would be sure to try to use all of the skills he had learned in treatment. He added, however, that he would definitely reach out if he ever thought he was in danger of relapsing. At this point, we ended the session and said our good-byes.

# CHAPTER 16

# Conclusion

We've come a long way in our understanding and treatment of OCD since Jean-Étienne Dominique Esquirol first described OCD in the psychiatric literature in 1838. Yet, we still have much more work to do. Despite our best efforts, OCD remains the fourth most common mental disorder after depression, alcohol/substance misuse, and social phobia (Kessler et al., 2005) and is ranked by the World Health Organization as one of the 10 most handicapping conditions by lost income and decreased quality of life (Bobes et al., 2001). In addition, the International OCD Foundation (IOCDF) notes that, on average, people with OCD see three to four doctors and spend 9 years seeking treatment before they receive a correct diagnosis, and that it takes an average of 17 years from the time OCD begins for people to obtain appropriate treatment.

Part of this delay has historically been linked to patient factors, such as people with OCD being secretive and attempting to hide their symptoms, often out of shame and fear of stigma. Another part of the delay has historically been linked to a general lack of public awareness of OCD, leaving many people suffering from OCD unaware that their symptoms were actually part of a treatable disorder. Fortunately, an increase in mainstream media attention to OCD in recent years seems to have benefited sufferers by addressing both of these factors via an increase in awareness and destigmatization. It should be emphasized, however, that many forms of OCD are less "classic" or common and therefore may not be so easily recognized by the person, the person's family, friends, or coworkers—or even by health care providers. As such, more work needs to be done to increase the familiarity of primary care physicians (PCPs) with OCD symptoms, as they are often the first line of defense against the disorder, and a lack of awareness and understanding of the symptoms can lead to the wrong diagnosis and failure to provide or refer to appropriate treatments.

The good news is that we now have several effective treatment options for OCD. The expert consensus guidelines (e.g., March et al., 1997; National Institute for Health and Clinical Excellence, 2005; Nathan & Gorman, 2007; www.psychologicaltreatments.org) consistently suggest that of the many different psychological treatments offered for OCD, Ex/RP has the strongest evidence base. Most guidelines recommend either starting treatment with Ex/RP alone or in combination with a medication, depending on factors such as the severity of the OCD and the age of the patient. Most studies show that, on average, about 70% of patients with OCD will benefit from Ex/RP and/or a medication, with patients who respond to Ex/RP on average reporting a 60–80% reduction in OCD symptoms and patients on medicine usually reporting a 40–60% reduction in

OCD symptoms. Patients, however, must actively participate in CBT, and medicines have to be taken consistently and as prescribed in order for the treatments to work. Unfortunately, studies show that at least 25% of patients with OCD refuse CBT, and as many as half of patients with OCD discontinue medicines owing to side effects or for other reasons.

Given all of these facts, here are a few final take-home messages for you to consider. First, it is important to understand and remember just how difficult it can be to treat patients suffering from OCD. Remember that by the time a patient with OCD reaches your office, he will, on average, have been suffering with the symptoms for more than a decade and a half and will have spent roughly half of that time seeking appropriate treatment—only to find that he does not get it—despite several attempts. During this time, he may also be struggling to hide his worsening symptoms, out of either shame or fear, and his symptoms may cause him to struggle at work, at home, and in his social life. In short, by the time the average patient with OCD finds you for treatment, he may have been struggling with his symptoms for many years, without any relief, despite seeking help. And he may have lost hope.

As such, it is important to remember to spend time building (and then maintaining) a trusting alliance and collaborative relationship with your patients. Part of this alliance will no doubt be built when you and your patient agree on your goals and tasks. However, another part of this alliance is built when patients feel a bond to their therapists (i.e., believe their therapist understands them and cares about them). Remember, you're about to embark on a journey together during which time you'll be asking them to face some of their worst fears. If they don't believe they can trust in the treatment (or you), they may decide it is not for them.

By now, it should be clear that the treatment to start with for OCD is Ex/RP (and possibly, medications). However, it should also be clear that before diving in with the treatment, it is critical that you first conduct a thorough diagnostic and clinical evaluation and then create a comprehensive case formulation for each patient. This will allow you to customize the treatment plan for OCD outlined in this book to fit each patient's idiosyncratic symptoms, history, culture, context, and so on—rather than force each patient to fit into a particular treatment protocol.

The case formulation and treatment plan should then be revisited often and revised whenever necessary—especially if the patient's symptoms or life circumstances shift or if treatment gains are not being made (or held). All too often, clinicians facing plateaus in treatment simply opt to continue what they've been doing rather than try to problem-solve how to improve the outcome. At certain times this may call for adjustments to be made in the core Ex/RP treatment; at other times it may call for a change in direction—for example, to move to motivation-enhancing techniques or to one or more the supplementary treatment techniques from cognitive therapy, ACT, or metacognitive therapy; and at yet other times, it may call for a good referral to be made to a trusted colleague.

Remember, the comprehensive treatment plan detailed in this book, along with the supplementary techniques and tools it describes, are all meant to expand your understanding of OCD and help build your clinical "tool box" of techniques to draw on—if and when you deem them to be appropriate to try with a particular patient reporting specific symptoms, under specific circumstances. With a different patient, the "recipe for success" will likely need different ingredients. Ultimately, however, it is up to you to use your best clinical judgment when conceptualizing a case and planning treatment interventions. I wish you all the best in your clinical endeavors with this highly challenging but extremely rewarding population.

# Resources

# ADDITIONAL READING FOR PROFESSIONALS

*Clinical Obsessive–Compulsive Disorders in Adults and Children* by Robert Hudak and Darin D. Dougherty (Cambridge University Press, 2011).

*Cognitive-Behavioral Therapy for OCD* by David A. Clark (Guilford Press, 2004).

*Cognitive-Behavioral Treatment of Childhood OCD: It's Only a False Alarm—Therapist Guide* by John Piacentini, Audra Langley and Tami Roblek (Oxford University Press, 2007).

*Cognitive Therapy for Obsessive–Compulsive Disorder: A Guide for Professionals* by Sabine Wilhelm and Gail S. Steketee (New Harbinger, 2006).

*Exposure and Response (Ritual) Prevention for Obsessive–Compulsive Disorder: Therapist Guide* by Edna B. Foa, Elna Yadin, and Tracey K. Lichner (Oxford University Press, 2012).

*Family-Based Treatment for Young Children with OCD: Therapist Guide* by Jennifer B. Freeman and Abbe Marrs Garcia (Oxford University Press, 2009).

*Handbook of Child and Adolescent Obsessive–Compulsive Disorder* edited by Eric A. Storch, Gary R. Geffken, and Tanya K. Murphy (Erlbaum, 2007).

*Mastery of Obsessive–Compulsive Disorder: Therapist Guide* by Michael J. Kozak and Edna B. Foa (Oxford University Press, 1997).

*Obsessive–Compulsive Disorder* by Jonathan S. Abramowitz (Hogrefe, 2006).

*OCD in Children and Adolescents: A Cognitive-Behavioral Treatment Manual* by John S. March and Karen Mulle (Guilford Press, 1998).

*Overcoming Obsessive–Compulsive Disorder: Therapist Protocol* by Gail S. Steketee (New Harbinger, 1999).

*Psychological Treatment of Obsessive–Compulsive Disorder: Fundamentals and Beyond* edited by Martin M. Antony, Christine Purdon, and Laura J. Summerfeldt (American Psychological Association, 2007).

*Treatment of Obsessive–Compulsive Disorder* by Lata K. McGinn and William C. Sanderson (Jason Aronson, 1999).

*Treatment of Obsessive Compulsive Disorder* by Gail Steketee (Guilford Press, 1993).

# ADDITIONAL READING FOR PATIENTS

*A Thought Is Just a Thought: A Story of Living with OCD* by Leslie Talley (Lantern Books, 2006).

*Coping with OCD: Practical Strategies for Living Well with Obsessive–Compulsive Disorder* by Bruce M. Hyman and Troy DuFrene (New Harbinger, 2008).

*Freedom from Obsessive–Compulsive Disorder: A Personalized Recovery Program for Living with Uncertainty* by Jonathan Grayson (Penguin, 2014).

*Freeing Your Child from Obsessive–Compulsive Disorder: A Powerful, Practical Program for Parents of Children and Adolescents* by Tamar E. Chansky (Harmony, 2001).

*Getting Over OCD: A 10-Step Workbook for Taking Back Your Life* by Jonathan S. Abramowitz (Guilford Press, 2009).

*Kissing Doorknobs* by Terry Spencer Hesser (Random House, 1998).

*Mastery of Obsessive–Compulsive Disorder: Client Workbook* by Edna B. Foa and Michael J. Kozak (Oxford University Press, 1997).

*The Mindfulness Workbook for OCD: A Guide to Overcoming Obsessions and Compulsions Using Mindfulness and Cognitive Behavioral Therapy* by Jon Hershfield and Tom Corboy (New Harbinger, 2013).

*OCD: A Guide for the Newly Diagnosed* by Michael A. Tompkins (New Harbinger, 2012).

*The OCD Answer Book: Professional Answers to More Than 250 Top Questions about Obsessive–Compulsive Disorder* by Patrick B. McGrath (Sourcebooks, 2007).

*The OCD Workbook: Your Guide to Breaking Free from Obsessive–Compulsive Disorder* by Bruce M. Hyman and Cherry Pedrick (New Harbinger, 2010).

*Out of the Rabbit Hole: A Road Map to Freedom from OCD* by Sheri Bloom and Suzanne Mouton-Odum (Wonderland Press, 2013).

*Overcoming Obsessive–Compulsive Disorder: Client Manual* by Gail S. Steketee (New Harbinger, 1999).

*Overcoming Obsessive Thoughts: How to Gain Control of Your OCD* by Christine Purdon and David A. Clark (New Harbinger, 2005).

*Stop Obsessing!: How to Overcome Your Obsessions and Compulsions (Revised Edition)* by Edna B. Foa and Reid Wilson (Bantam Books, 2001).

*Take Control of OCD: The Ultimate Guide for Kids with OCD* by Bonnie Zucker (Prufrock Press, 2011),

*Talking Back to OCD: The Program That Helps Kids and Teens Say "No Way"—and Parents Say "Way to Go"* by John S. March with Christine M. Benton (Guilford Press, 2007).

*Treating Your OCD with Exposure and Response (Ritual) Prevention: Workbook* by Elna Yadin, Edna B. Foa, and Tracey K. Lichner (Oxford University Press, 2012).

*What to Do When Your Brain Gets Stuck: A Kid's Guide to Overcoming OCD* by Dawn Huebner (Magination Press, 2007).

*What to Do When Your Child Has Obsessive–Compulsive Disorder: Strategies and Solutions* by Aureen Pinto Wagner (Lighthouse Press, 2002).

*When in Doubt, Make Belief: An OCD-Inspired Approach to Living with Uncertainty* by Jeff Bell (New World Library, 2009).

## HELPFUL WEBSITES

**American Academy of Child and Adolescent Psychiatry (AACAP)**
Facts for Families: OCD in Children and Adolescents
*www.aacap.org/AACAP/Families_and_Youth/Facts_for_Families/FFF-Guide/Obsessive-Compulsive-Disorder-In-Children-And-Adolescents-060.aspx*

**American Psychiatric Association (APA)**
*www.psychiatry.org/patients-families/ocd*

**Anxieties.com**
*http://anxieties.com/94/ocd*

**Anxiety Disorders Association of British Columbia (AnxietyBC)**
*www.anxietybc.com*

**Anxiety and Depression Association of America (ADAA)**
*www.adaa.org/understanding-anxiety/obsessive-compulsive-disorder-ocd*

**Association for Behavioral and Cognitive Therapies (ABCT)**
*www.abct.org*

**Beyondblue**
*www.beyondblue.org.au/the-facts/anxiety/types-of-anxiety/ocd*

**Beyond OCD**
*http://beyondocd.org*

**Centre for Addiction and Mental Health (CAMH)**
*www.camh.ca/en/hospital/health_information/a_z_mental_health_and_addiction_information/*
    *obsessive_compulsive_disorder/obsessive_compulsive_disorder_information_guide/Pages/*
    *obsessive_compulsive_disorder_information_guide.aspx*

**Helpguide**
*www.helpguide.org/articles/anxiety/obssessive-compulsive-disorder-ocd.htm*

**International OCD Foundation (IOCDF)**
*https://iocdf.org*

**Kids Health—Kids**
*http://kidshealth.org/kid/feeling/emotion/ocd.html*

**Kids Health—Parents**
*http://kidshealth.org/parent/emotions/behavior/OCD.html*

**Mayo Clinic**
*www.mayoclinic.org/diseases-conditions/ocd/basics/definition/con-20027827*

**National Alliance on Mental Illness (NAMI)**
*www.nami.org/Learn-More/Mental-Health-Conditions/Obsessive-Compulsive-Disorder*

**National Institute of Mental Health (NIMH)**
Obsessive–Compulsive Disorder
*www.nimh.nih.gov/health/topics/obsessive-compulsive-disorder-ocd/index.shtml*

**NHS Choices**
Obsessive Compulsive Disorder (OCD)
*www.nhs.uk/conditions/obsessive-compulsive-disorder/Pages/Introduction.aspx*

**OCD Action**
*www.ocdaction.org.uk*

**OCD Challenge**
*https://ocdchallenge.com*

**OCD Ireland**
*www.ocdireland.org*

**OCD Resource Center of Florida**
*www.ocdhope.com*

**OCD-UK**
*www.ocduk.org*

**Patient: Trusted Medical Information and Support**
*http://patient.info/health/obsessive-compulsive-disorder-leaflet*

**PsychCentral**
Obsessive–Compulsive Disorder
*http://psychcentral.com/disorders/ocd*

**WebMD**
*www.webmd.com/mental-health/obsessive-compulsive-disorder*

**Womenshealth.gov**
*www.womenshealth.gov/mental-health/illnesses/obsessive-compulsive-disorder.html*

**Yahoo Health Groups**
The OCD and Parenting List
*https://groups.yahoo.com/neo/groups/ocdandparenting/info*


## SOURCES FOR EXPERT CONSENSUS GUIDELINES FOR THE TREATMENT OF OCD

**Clinical Guidelines CG31: Obsessive Compulsive Disorder (OCD)
    and Body Dysmorphic Disorder (BDD)**
from the National Institute for Health and Clinical Excellence
*www.nice.org.uk/guidance/CG31*

**Evidence-Based Treatment for Children and Adolescents**
from Division 53 of the American Psychological Association
*http://effectivechildtherapy.org*

**Living with OCD from PsychGuides**
*www.psychguides.com/guides/living-with-ocd-obsessive-compulsive-disorder*

**Obsessive–Compulsive Disorder: When Unwanted Thoughts Take Over**
from the National Institute of Mental Health
*www.nimh.nih.gov/health/publications/obsessive-compulsive-disorder-when-unwanted-thoughts-take-over/
    index.shtml*

**Practice Guideline for the Treatment of Patients with Obsessive–Compulsive Disorder**
from the Agency for Healthcare Research and Quality
*www.guidelines.gov/content.aspx?id=11078*

**Research-Supported Psychological Treatments**
from Division 12 of the American Psychological Association
*www.divl2.org/psychological-treatments*

**Treatment of Patients with Obsessive–Compulsive Disorder**
from the American Psychiatric Association
*http://psychiatryonline.org/pb/assets/raw/sitewide/practice_guidelines/guidelines/ocd.pdf*

## EMPIRICALLY BASED MEASURES FOR OCD AND RELATED CONSTRUCTS

Brown Assessment of Beliefs Scale
Child Obsessive Compulsive Impact Scale
Children's Measure of Obsessive–Compulsive Symptoms
Children's Obsessional Compulsive Inventory
Children's Yale–Brown Obsessive–Compulsive Scale—Child Report and Parent Report
Clark–Beck Obsessive–Compulsive Inventory
Compulsive Activity Checklist
Dimensional Obsessive–Compulsive Scale
Dimensional Yale–Brown Obsessive Compulsive Inventory
Florida Obsessive–Compulsive Inventory
Florida Obsessive–Compulsive Student Inventory
Frost Indecisiveness Scale
Hamburg Obsession/Compulsion Inventory—Short Form
Interpretations of Intrusions Inventory
Intolerance of Uncertainty Scale
Leyton Obsessional Inventory
Maudsley Obsessional Compulsive Inventory
Meta-Cognitions Questionnaire
Multidimensional Perfectionism Scale
National Institute of Mental Health Global Obsessive–Compulsive Scale
National Institute of Mental Health Obsessive–Compulsive Rating Scale
Obsessive Beliefs Questionnaire
Obsessive–Compulsive Inventory
Obsessive–Compulsive Inventory—Revised
Overvalued Ideation Scale
Padua Inventory—Revised
Padua Inventory—Palatine Revision
Padua Inventory—Washington State University Revision
Partner Related Obsessive Compulsive Symptom Inventory
Relationship Obsessive Compulsive Inventory
Responsibility Attitudes Questionnaire
Responsibility Interpretations Questionnaire
Saving Inventory—Revised
Schedule of Compulsions, Obsessions, and Pathological Impulses
Self-Rated Scale for Obsessive–Compulsive Disorder
Symmetry, Ordering, and Arranging Questionnaire

Thought–Action Fusion Scale
Thought Control Questionnaire
Vancouver Obsessional Compulsive Inventory
Vancouver Obsessional Compulsive Inventory—Revised
Yale–Brown Obsessive–Compulsive Inventory
Yale–Brown Obsessive–Compulsive Scale—Self-Report

# Reproducible Forms

# FORM 1.  Phone Screen Template

Date contacted: _____

Date of Screen: _____

Name: _____ Age: _____

Phone number: _____ OK to leave a message?  Y/N

Referral source: _____

Current symptoms: _____

Patient's ratings of symptom severity:

Current (1–10): _____ Best in past year (1–10): _____ Worst in past year (1–10): _____

Previous treatment(s)?  Y/N

Helpful?  Y/N   Why or why not? _____

Tried CBT in past?  Y/N

Current risk factors:

Using drugs/alcohol:  Y/N

Suicidal/homicidal ideation:  Y/N

Other factors that may impact treatment:

Support from friends and/or family:  Y/N

Time/scheduling/transportation/distance constraints:  Y/N

Motivation to change (0–10): _____ Readiness to Change (0–10): _____

Psychoeducational materials provided

Brief overview of CBT:  Y/N

Brief overview of typical course of treatment:  Y/N

Office hours, fees, appointment policies?  Y/N

Appointment scheduled:  Y/N

If yes, scheduled for (date/time): _____

Gave patient address and directions?  Y/N

If no, reason: _____

Gave patient alternative referrals?  Y/N

Notes or comments: _____

_____

# FORM 2.  Decisional Balance Worksheet

**Instructions:** When we think about making changes, most of us don't really consider all "sides" in a complete way. Instead we often do what we think we "should" do, avoid doing those things we don't feel like doing, or just feel confused or overwhelmed and give up thinking about it at all. Thinking through the pros and cons of both changing and not making a change is one way to help us make sure we have fully considered a possible change. This can help us to "hang on" to our plan in times of stress or frustration. Below, write in the reasons that you can think of in each of the boxes.

| | Benefits/Pros (Short-term and long-term) | Costs/Cons (Short-term and long-term) |
|---|---|---|
| **Do not make a change** (e.g., "Do not give Ex/RP a try and continue to manage my OCD the same way I always have.") | | |
| **Make a change** (e.g., "Give Ex/RP a try so I can learn to manage my OCD in new way.") | | |

# FORM 3. Common Questions and Answers about OCD

For many patients, entering into treatment is a big step and comes with a lot of questions. This handout is designed to provide you with answers to the most common questions that patients have about their OCD. If you need more information or you have a question that is not answered on this handout, please be sure to bring it up with your therapist.

### Question: Can I expect to fully eliminate my OCD?

*Answer:* No! It is *normal* for most people to experience some *symptoms* of OCD. Experiencing symptoms of OCD does not mean you have a disorder! Symptoms only become a disorder when they cause a lot of (1) distress, (2) disruption, and/or (3) disability in your work, home, or social life. As a result, the goal of treatment is to help you learn how to manage your OCD symptoms more effectively. The research suggests that on average, you can expect a 60–70% improvement in your symptom severity if you fully participate in and complete the treatment.

### Question: Is homework really necessary?

*Answer:* Yes! CBT is unlike other types of talk therapy for this very reason. In CBT the assigning of homework is seen as essential in order for you to (1) practice building the skills you are taught in each session, (2) gather evidence to test out predictions you make in each session, (3) demonstrate that the same rules apply to life inside and outside of your therapist's office, and (4) help you learn to do the treatment on your own—without the aid of your therapist. The research is strong here: if you do not complete your homework assignments, you will not do as well in this treatment.

### Question: The CBT model seems too simple! Isn't OCD more complicated than that?

*Answer:* Perhaps the model seems simple, and yes, there are many competing theories about what causes and maintains OCD. But the model does not have to be complex to be effective. And simple does not mean easy. Psychological change requires two big things: insight and awareness into the problem and a willingness and commitment to do what it takes to change it. While CBT takes a simple approach, breaking down what you need to focus on into two main categories (find a new way to deal with your thoughts and change what you've been doing in response to your triggers), it still takes a while to learn how to spot your triggers, understand how your reactions andinterpretations of the triggers generate your anxiety, and realize when you're engaging in rituals. It takes a great deal of courage and conviction to break the cycle.

### Question: Is full ritual prevention really necessary? Can't I just keep a couple of them?

*Answer:* Yes, full ritual prevention is really necessary. To engage in partial ritual prevention is a bit like working hard to throw buckets of water on a fire, only to throw on the occasional jug of gasoline: in the end, the fire will keep on burning! Or think of it like removing the weeds in a garden. If you leave one or two weeds, it's only a matter of time before they start to take over again. In other words, at best, engaging in occasional rituals can dampen the impact of the treatment and prolong it unnecessarily, and at worst, engaging in occasional rituals can interfere with the new learning that is necessary to change the way you see your symptoms and set you up for a potential relapse after treatment is terminated. If you really want to maintain some of your rituals, it may mean that you have

*(cont.)*

not fully understood the CBT model or treatment explanation, or that you have some special rules for certain triggers or thoughts, or are still not quite sure whether this treatment is right for you. If this is the case, you should speak with your therapist about it before starting the treatment.

### Question: Surely some of my fears are based in reality?

*Answer:* Of course! The themes of the fearsome thoughts that people with OCD experience have been found to be the *exact same* as those experienced by people who do not have OCD. The only difference is that people with OCD experience these fearsome thoughts much more frequently, intensely, and for longer periods of time. This happens because people with OCD often interpret these houghts in ways that people without OCD do not. For example, people with OCD cannot seem to tolerate the uncertainty about which fears are based in reality and which are not as well as people without OCD. The treatment aims at correcting this intolerance of uncertainty through Ex/RP. By exposing yourself to your fears while preventing yourself from engaging in the rituals that are often performed to create more certainty (e.g., checking to make sure the stove is turned off) you will gradually learn to tolerate uncertainty more and more and you will not need to ritualize in order to feel better. This is why facing your fears and learning to tolerate your anxious feelings are necessary component of this treatment.

### Question: Are you sure nothing bad will happen (to me or my loved ones) if I do this treatment?

*Answer:* Yes and no. Although this treatment has been studies for many years in patients around the world with OCD and has been recommended as the treatment of choice for OCD by experts in the fields of psychiatry and psychology, you can never *guarantee* that bad things won't happen in life. In fact, it is quite the opposite: eventually bad things happen in *all* of our lives—and so instead of spending so much of your time and effort trying to avoid thoughts about them or prevent them from happening, you must learn a *new way* to deal with your thoughts about them. This treatment will help you to *test out* whether your rituals are really preventing bad things from happening and to feel more confident in your ability to determine when something is actually posing a serious threat to you or a loved one.

### Question: How certain are you that I will see a positive result?

*Answer:* It depends on what is meant by a positive result. As was mentioned above, the research suggests that on average, you can expect a 60–70% improvement in your symptom severity if you fully complete the treatment. But it's really more than just completing the treatment: one of the biggest factors in maximizing the results is the amount of work you do in each session as well as between the sessions to develop the skills necessary to become your own CBT therapist.

### Question: Have you treated anyone like me before? From what I've read my symptoms don't seem common. Are you sure they will respond to this approach?

*Answer:* Just as no two people are the same, no two patients are exactly the same. There are more common symptoms and less common symptoms of OCD. However, even if the symptoms are not common and do not fit neatly into any of the classic themes, the power of the CBT model of OCD is in the fact that it can be used to explain how *any* symptom of OCD is maintained—which can lead to the appropriate and successful treatment of that symptom.

# FORM 4. Self-Monitoring Form

**Instructions:** It is very important to obtain accurate information about the frequency and duration of your obsessions and compulsions. This information can be used to increase your awareness of your triggers, monitor your progress, and, if necessary, adjust the treatment exercises. It can be difficult to self-monitor your symptoms, especially if you have a lot of them or are not used to paying attention to when they occur. This Self-Monitoring Form is designed to help you to capture this information in a simple, straightforward way (e.g., you do *not* need to write long paragraphs, but rather just a few words in each box). Please keep this form with you at *all times* and *immediately* complete an entry each *time* you engage in a ritual (do *not* save recording for later in the day, as it will not be as accurate and will not benefit you as much).

| **Trigger** for the obsession (or **situation** you were in when you experienced the obsession) | **Obsession** | **Interpretation** (what having the obsession means to you or says about you) | Level of **Anxiety or Discomfort it caused you** (0–10) | **Ritual/Compulsion** (what you did to feel better) | **Time** spent on the ritual (in minutes) or **number of times** you performed the ritual |
|---|---|---|---|---|---|
| | | | | | |
| | | | | | |
| | | | | | |
| | | | | | |
| | | | | | |
| | | | | | |
| | | | | | |

# FORM 5. Fact Sheet on Obsessive–Compulsive Disorder

The following facts on OCD have been provided by the National Institutes of Health (NIH). Often it is helpful to review it and return to your next session with a written summary of the main points and a written list of any questions that you have after reading it.

According to the 2005 National Comorbidity Survey-Replication study, about 2.2 million American adults have obsessive–compulsive disorder (OCD), a brain disorder that often begins in childhood. The persistent, unwanted thoughts and rituals of OCD sometimes take over people's lives to the point that they can't work or maintain relationships or engage in everyday tasks and social interactions.

## YESTERDAY

- The standard treatment for OCD was a type of long-term psychotherapy aimed at overcoming psychological defenses. There was no evidence that this treatment was effective.

- Clinicians lacked objective measurements that could help them accurately diagnose OCD—a crucial prerequisite for appropriate treatment.

- There were no proven medications for OCD.

- OCD was thought of primarily as a psychoanalytic issue, not a brain disorder.

## TODAY

- Effective treatments are now available. Among them are antidepressant medications that act on serotonin, one of several neurotransmitters (brain chemicals) through which brain cells communicate with each other. These medications also act on brain systems and circuits involved in OCD. Recently developed antipsychotic medications may become another option when prescribed alongside standard medications for hard-to-treat patients with OCD.

- A type of psychotherapy called "exposure and response prevention," which breaks the cycle of repetitive behavior, is an effective treatment for many patients.

- Clinicians now have objective tools for identifying OCD subtypes and measuring their severity, allowing treatment to be personalized.

- Imaging studies show that people with OCD have differences in specific brain areas, compared with other people. Successfully treated patients have brain-activity patterns like those of healthy people.

- Traditionally, OCD was thought to "run in families." Genetic studies now suggest that variations in certain genes are involved and that risk is higher when certain variations occur together.

- Researchers are following up on early evidence that infection from the *Streptococcus* bacterium might lead to some cases of OCD.

- Using genetic engineering, NIH-funded researchers created an OCD-like set of behaviors in mice. They then reversed these behaviors with antidepressants and genetic targeting of a key brain circuit. The study suggests new strategies for treating the disorder.

*(cont.)*

## TOMORROW

- Researchers are studying the potential of deep-brain stimulation, a surgical technique that stimulates cells in specific brain areas, for patients who don't respond to other treatments.

- Genetics research may help clinicians decide what treatments are likely to work for each patient. Whether a treatment works may be partly due to variations in certain genes.

- Imaging, molecular biology, and genetics research are pointing the way to brain mechanisms involved in OCD. Features of these mechanisms are potential biomarkers that could identify people at risk—a key to early intervention.

- Research to identify brain mechanisms involved in OCD also holds the potential to reveal targets for better medications with fewer side effects.

For more information, please contact the NIMH Information Center at *nimhinfo@nih.gov* or 301-443-4513.

National Institute of Mental Health (NIMH) *www.nimh.nih.gov.*

# FORM 6.   Chart for Recording Check on OCD Symptoms

**Instructions:** At the start of each session, you should have the patient provide subjective ratings, using an average from 0 to 10, for severity of the OCD symptoms, amount of effort put into the treatment, and success in managing the OCD symptoms since the last session. You can then use this information (graphing is ideal) to provide the patient with immediate feedback on how the patient is progressing in treatment. You can also examine the ratings together and look for connections between effort, success/control, and overall OCD symptom severity.

| Session Number | OCD Severity | Effort | Success/Managing |
|:---:|:---:|:---:|:---:|
| 1 | | | |
| 2 | | | |
| 3 | | | |
| 4 | | | |
| 5 | | | |
| 6 | | | |
| 7 | | | |
| 8 | | | |
| 9 | | | |
| 10 | | | |
| 11 | | | |
| 12 | | | |
| 13 | | | |
| 14 | | | |
| 15 | | | |
| 16 | | | |

# FORM 7.  A CBT Model of OCD

Below is a CBT model that explains how OCD is maintained and can even worsen over time. As you can see below, certain situations and triggers generate intrusive thoughts which, if appraised and interpreted in certain problematic ways, can go on to become obsessions and generate intense feelings of anxiety. This often leads people to engage in rituals (compulsions) in order to decrease the anxiety they are feeling. While performing rituals may work in the short term, in the long term it only works against you, as each time a ritual is performed, the relief you feel serves to strengthen the connection between the obsession and ritual that "needs" to be performed in order to feel relief ("If it worked last time, there must be something to it!"). In addition, as the connection between the obsession and ritual is strengthened, the situations, triggers, thoughts, and appraisals all become more important—which makes you look out for them even more . . . and notice them more frequently! This then leads to more constant feelings of anxiety, which leads to more rituals, and the like.

See if you can apply the model to your own cycle of OCD.

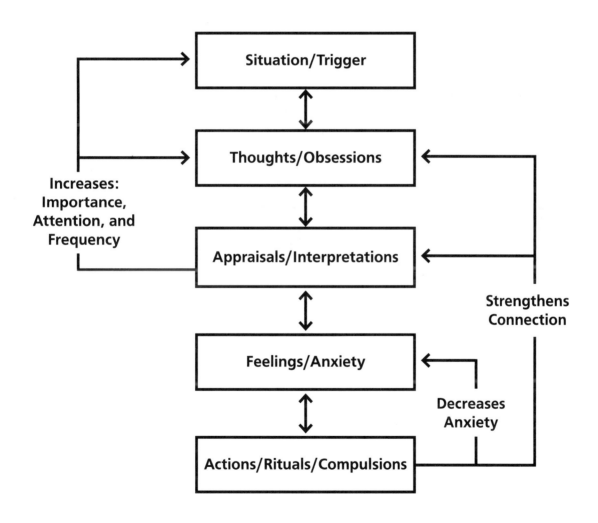

# FORM 8. Subjective Units of Distress Scale (SUDS)

Everybody experiences anxiety at times, but what makes one person anxious may not make another person anxious. For example, while watching a scary movie in a theater some people will scream out loud and/or cover their eyes during a certain scene, while other people watching the same scene might not feel so scared, and still others might find the same scene boring (especially if they have seen it before!).

Unfortunately, unlike other areas of medicine that are able to assess for problems using blood tests or X-rays, there are no simple tests available for measuring a person's level of distress. As a result, cognitive-behavioral therapists often have their patients create and use a **Subjective Units of Distress Scale ("SUDS")** in order to help them quantify and communicate the level of anxiety they experience during exposure exercises. Note that while the term "distress" is often used to refer to feelings of anxiety, it really can apply to *any negative emotional state* (e.g., anger, fear, upset).

In the case of OCD, creating a SUDS allows therapists to measure each patient's reaction to various situations, triggers, and obsessions. The scale range typically runs from 0 to 10, although some patients feel more comfortable using a 0 to 100 scale. Either way is fine. Note that a rating of 0 is meant to represent *no distress at all* (i.e., completely calm, relaxed), while a rating of 10 (or 100) is meant to represent *very extreme distress*—often to the point of experiencing panic-like symptoms or even full-scale panic attacks.

It is also helpful to identify some specific situations, ideally those that are fairly recent and unrelated to your OCD, that correspond with different SUDS ratings for you. These are referred to as "anchor points" because they "anchor" the SUDS by linking real experiences from your life to the 0, midway, and 10-point levels on the scale. These can then be used throughout treatment to compare the level of SUDS that an exposure item generates versus these anchor points in your past. Your therapist will help you identify these anchor points and record them on a form called a SUDS Template for you to review.

*(cont.)*

**SUDS TEMPLATE**

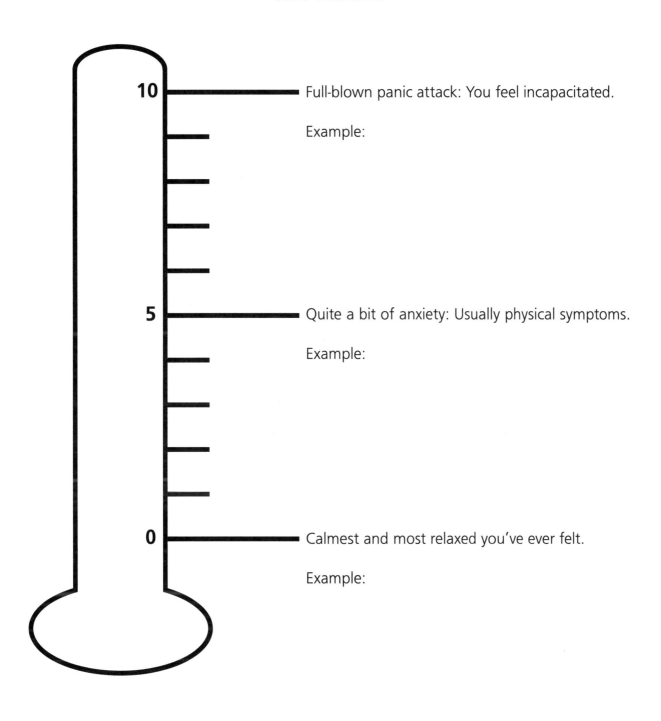

10    Full-blown panic attack: You feel incapacitated.

Example:

5    Quite a bit of anxiety: Usually physical symptoms.

Example:

0    Calmest and most relaxed you've ever felt.

Example:

# FORM 9.  Hierarchy Construction Worksheet

**Instructions:** This worksheet provides a template for identifying and rating anxiety-provoking items that can then be used to create a hierarchy for Ex/RP. Begin by generating a list of anxiety-producing items. Next, have the patient rate the severity of anxiety that each item on the list produces using his or her SUDS. Finally, sort the items from highest to lowest anxiety, noting the date the ratings were obtained. Reuse this worksheet at certain points during the course of treatment to add new items and/or assess whether the original items are becoming less anxiety-provoking.

| Item | SUDS (Date:         ) | SUDS (Date:         ) | SUDS (Date:         ) | SUDS (Date:         ) |
|------|------|------|------|------|
|      |      |      |      |      |
|      |      |      |      |      |
|      |      |      |      |      |
|      |      |      |      |      |
|      |      |      |      |      |
|      |      |      |      |      |
|      |      |      |      |      |
|      |      |      |      |      |
|      |      |      |      |      |
|      |      |      |      |      |
|      |      |      |      |      |
|      |      |      |      |      |
|      |      |      |      |      |
|      |      |      |      |      |
|      |      |      |      |      |
|      |      |      |      |      |
|      |      |      |      |      |

# FORM 10. Ex/RP Practice Record

**Instructions:** The form on the following page should be used **each time** you complete an exposure practice.

First, record the date and then briefly note the item, situation, or imaginal scenario from your hierarchy that you are using for the exposure practice.

Next, record the time you start the exposure practice, as well as the time you end it.

**Before starting**: note your **current** SUDS level where it says "Pre-SUDS (Anticipatory Anxiety)", as well as how high you **predict** your SUDS will get where it says "Predicted Max SUDS," along with what you **fear** will happen (be specific!), and how **strongly** you belief your prediction.

**After starting:** rate your SUDS immediately after starting your exposure practice ("SUDS at start") and then at 10-minute intervals throughout the exposure practice—ideally until your initial SUDS are reduced by approximately 50% or more.

**After finishing:** note your SUDS as well as the maximum level you reached during the exposure practice ("Max SUDS"), report the results of your feared prediction and how strongly you believe it after finishing the practice, and list any alternative beliefs you have developed about the feared outcome, along with a rating of how strongly you belief them. Finally, rate how strong your urge to ritualize is, as well as how willing you are to engage in ritual prevention.

Be sure to add comments about this exposure practice in the space left at the bottom of the form! Especially anything new that you learned and any difficulties that you encountered—either during the exposure or after finishing it.

*(cont.)*

## EX/RP PRACTICE RECORD

**Name:** _____  **Date:** _____

Exposure item/situation/imaginal scenario: _____

Exposure start time: _____  Exposure end time: _____

Pre-SUDS (Anticipatory Anxiety): _____  Predicted Max. SUDS: _____

Feared outcome and/or consequences (be specific!): _____

_____

_____

Strength of belief in feared outcome before starting (0–10): _____

SUDS at start: _____  SUDS at 10 minutes: _____  SUDS at 20 minutes: _____  SUDS at 30 minutes: _____

SUDS at 40 minutes: _____  SUDS after 50 minutes: _____  SUDS at end: _____  Max. SUDS: _____

Results of feared outcome: _____  Belief in feared outcome at end (0–10): _____

Alternative beliefs about the feared outcome and/or consequences: _____

_____

_____

Strength of belief in alternative beliefs (0–10): _____

Urge to ritualize at end (0–10): _____  Willingness to engage in ritual prevention (0–10): _____

Comments about this practice, including anything new that was learned and any difficulties that were encountered: _____

_____

_____

***Congratulations for doing the exposure practice!***

***While it can be very challenging to complete, it is an important step in maximizing your treatment outcome.***

# Obsessive–Compulsive Inventory—Revised (OCI-R)

# FORM 11. Obsessive–Compulsive Inventory—Revised (OCI-R)

**Instructions:** The following statements refer to experiences that many people have in their everyday lives. Circle the number that best describes **HOW MUCH** that experience has **DISTRESSED or BOTHERED you during the PAST MONTH**. The numbers refer to the following verbal labels:

0 = Not at all     1 = A little     2 = Moderately     3 = A lot     4 = Extremely

**1.** I have saved up so many things that they get in the way.     0  1  2  3  4

**2.** I check things more often than necessary.     0  1  2  3  4

**3.** I get upset if objects are not arranged properly.     0  1  2  3  4

**4.** I feel compelled to count while I am doing things.     0  1  2  3  4

**5.** I find it difficult to touch an object when I know it has been touched by strangers or certain people.     0  1  2  3  4

**6.** I find it difficult to control my own thoughts.     0  1  2  3  4

**7.** I collect things I don't need.     0  1  2  3  4

**8.** I repeatedly check doors, windows, drawers, etc.     0  1  2  3  4

**9.** I get upset if others change the way I have arranged things.     0  1  2  3  4

**10.** I feel I have to repeat certain numbers.     0  1  2  3  4

**11.** I sometimes have to wash or clean myself simply because I feel contaminated.     0  1  2  3  4

**12.** I am upset by unpleasant thoughts that come into my mind against my will.     0  1  2  3  4

**13.** I avoid throwing things away because I am afraid I might need them later.     0  1  2  3  4

**14.** I repeatedly check gas and water taps and light switches after turning them off.     0  1  2  3  4

**15.** I need things to be arranged in a particular order.     0  1  2  3  4

**16.** I feel that there are good and bad numbers.     0  1  2  3  4

**17.** I wash my hands more often and longer than necessary.     0  1  2  3  4

**18.** I frequently get nasty thoughts and have difficulty in getting rid of them.     0  1  2  3  4

From "The Obsessive-Compulsive Inventory: Development and Validation of a Short Version" by Edna B. Foa et al. Copyright © 2002 American Psychological Association. Reprinted by permission.

## ADMINISTRATION AND SCORING

The OCI-R (Foa, Huppert, Leiberg, Langner, Kichic, Hajcak, & Salkovskis, 2002) is a short version of the OCI (Foa, Kozak, Salkovskis, Coles, & Amir, 1998). It is a self-report scale for assessing symptoms of OCD. It consists of 18 questions that a patient rates on a 5-point Likert scale.

The total score is obtained by adding the scores from all 18 items. The possible range of scores is 0–72. The mean score for patients with OCD is 28.0 ($SD$ = 13.53). The recommended cutoff score is 21, with scores at or above this level indicating the likely presence of OCD.

There are also six subscales built into the OCR-R. The scale item numbers are as follows:

> **Hoarding:** items 1, 7, 13
>
> **Checking:** items 2, 8, 14
>
> **Ordering:** items 3, 9, 15
>
> **Neutralizing:** items 4, 10, 16
>
> **Washing:** items 5, 11, 17
>
> **Obsessing:** items 6, 12, 18

The subscale scores are obtained by adding the scores of the respective items.

### References

Foa, E. B., Kozak, M. J., Salkovskis, P. M., Coles, M. E., & Amir, N. (1998). The validation of a new obsessive–compulsive disorder scale: The Obsessive–Compulsive Inventory. *Psychological Assessment, 10*(3), 206–214.

Foa, E. B., Huppert, J. D., Leiberg, S., Langner, R., Kichic, R., Hajcak, G., et al. (2002). The Obsessive–Compulsive Inventory: Development and validation of a short version. *Psychological Assessment, 14*(4), 485–496.

---

This Administration and Scoring section is to be used by the clinician and is *not* provided to the patient.

# References

Abramowitz, J. S. (1996). Variants of exposure and response prevention in the treatment of obsessive–compulsive disorder: A meta-analysis. *Behavior Therapy, 27,* 583–600.

Abramowitz, J. S. (2009). *Getting over OCD: A 10–step workbook for taking back your life.* New York: Guilford Press.

Abramowitz, J. [S.], & Houts, A. (2002). What is OCD and what is not? *Scientific Review of Mental Health Practice, 1*(2), 139–156.

American Psychiatric Association. (1952). *Diagnostic and statistical manual of mental disorders.* Washington, DC: Author.

American Psychiatric Association. (1968). *Diagnostic and statistical manual of mental disorders* (2nd ed.). Washington, DC: Author.

American Psychiatric Association. (1980). *Diagnostic and statistical manual of mental disorders* (3rd ed.). Washington, DC: Author.

American Psychiatric Association. (1987). *Diagnostic and statistical manual of mental disorders* (3rd ed., rev.). Washington, DC: Author.

American Psychiatric Association. (1994). *Diagnostic and statistical manual of mental disorders* (4th ed.). Washington, DC: Author.

American Psychiatric Association. (2000). *Diagnostic and statistical manual of mental disorders* (4th ed., text rev.). Washington, DC: Author.

American Psychiatric Association. (2013). *Diagnostic and statistical manual of mental disorders* (5th ed.). Arlington, VA: Author.

Antony, M. M., Orsillo, S. M., & Roemer, L. (2001). *Practitioner's guide to empirically-based measures of anxiety.* New York: Springer.

Arkowitz, H., Miller, W. R., & Rollnick, S. (Eds.). (2015). *Motivational interviewing in the treatment of psychological problems* (2nd ed.). New York: Guilford Press.

Barlow, D. H., Allen, L. B., & Choate, M. L. (2004). Toward a unified treatment for emotional disorders. *Behavior Therapy, 35*(2), 205–230.

Barr, L. C., Goodman, W. K., & Price, L. H. (1993). The serotonin hypothesis of obsessive compulsive disorder. *International Clinical Psychopharmacology, 8*(Suppl. 2), 79–82.

Beck, A. T. (1996). Beyond belief: A theory of modes, personality, and psychopathology. In P. M. Salkovskis (Ed.), *Frontiers of cognitive therapy* (pp. 1–25). New York; Guilford Press.

Beck, J. S. (2011). *Cognitive behavior therapy: Basics and beyond* (2nd ed.). New York; Guilford Press.

Bobes, J., Gonzalez, M. P., Bascaran, M. T., Arango, C., Saiz, P. A., & Bousono, M. (2001). Quality of life and disability in patients with obsessive–compulsive disorder. *European Psychiatry, 16,* 239–245.

Breiter, H. C., Rauch, S. L., Kwong, K. K., Baker, J. R., Weisskoff, R. M., Kennedy, D. N., et al. (1996). Functional magnetic resonance imaging of symptom provocation in obsessive–compulsive disorder. *Archives of General Psychiatry, 53*(7), 595.

Cottraux, J., Gérard, D., Cinotti, L., Froment, J. C., Deiber, M. P., Le Bars, D., et al. (1996). A controlled positron emission tomography study of obsessive and neutral auditory stimulation in obsessive–compulsive disorder with checking rituals. *Psychiatry Research, 60*(2), 101–112.

Cottraux, J., Yao, S. N., Lafont, S., Mollard, E., Bouvard, M., Sauteraud, A., et al. (2001). A randomized controlled trial of cognitive therapy versus intensive behavior therapy in obsessive compulsive disorder. *Psychotherapy and Psychosomatics, 70*(6), 288–297.

Craske, M. G., Liao, B., Brown, L., & Verliet, B. (2012). Role of inhibition in exposure therapy. *Journal of Experimental Psychopathology, 3*, 322–345.

Culver, N. C., Stoyanova, M., & Craske, M. G. (2012). Emotional variability and sustained arousal during exposure. *Journal of Behavior Therapy and Experimental Psychiatry, 43*(2), 787–793.

Denys, D., Zohar, J., & Westenberg, H. G. (2004). The role of dopamine in obsessive–compulsive disorder: Preclinical and clinical evidence. *Journal of Clinical Psychiatry, 65*, 11–17.

de Silva, P., & Marks, M. (1999). The role of traumatic experiences in the genesis of obsessive–compulsive disorder. *Behaviour Research and Therapy, 37*(10), 941–951.

Eisen, J. L., Phillips, K. A., Baer, L., Beer, D. A., Atala, K. D., & Rasmussen, S. A. (1998). The Brown Assessment of Beliefs Scale: Reliability and Validity. *American Journal of Psychiatry, 155*(1), 102–108.

Esquirol, J. E. D. (1838). *Des maladies mentales considérées sous les rapports médical hygiénique et médico-légal.* Paris: Baillière.

Fisher, P. L. (2009). Obsessive compulsive disorder: A comparison of CBT and the metacognitive approach. *International Journal of Cognitive Therapy, 2*(2), 107–122.

Fisher, P. L., & Wells, A. (2005). Experimental modification of beliefs in obsessive–compulsive disorder: A test of the metacognitive model. *Behaviour Research and Therapy, 43*(6), 821–829.

Flavell, J. H. (1979). Metacognition and cognitive monitoring: A new area of cognitive-developmental inquiry. *American Psychologist, 34*, 906–911.

Foa, E. B., Franklin, M. E., & Moser, J. (2002). Context in the clinic: How well do cognitive-behavioral therapies and medications work in combination? *Biological Psychiatry, 52*(10), 987–997.

Foa, E. B., Huppert, J. D., Leiberg, S., Langner, R., Kichic, R., Hajcak, G., et al. (2002). The Obsessive–Compulsive Inventory: Development and validation of a short version. *Psychological Assessment, 14*(4), 485–496.

Foa, E. B., & Kozak, M. J. (1995). DSM-IV field trial: Obsessive compulsive disorder. *American Journal of Psychiatry, 152*, 90–94.

Foa, E. B., Kozak, M. J., Salkovskis, P. M., Coles, M. E., & Amir, N. (1998). The validation of a new obsessive–compulsive disorder scale: The Obsessive–Compulsive Inventory. *Psychological Assessment, 10*(3), 206–214.

Foa, E. B., Liebowitz, M. R., Kozak, M. J., Davies, S., Campeas, R., Franklin, M. E., et al. (2005). Randomized, placebo-controlled trial of exposure and ritual prevention, clomipramine, and their combination in the treatment of obsessive–compulsive disorder. *American Journal of Psychiatry, 162*(1), 151–161.

Foa, E. B., & Wilson, R. (2009). *Stop obsessing!: How to overcome your obsessions and compulsions.* New York: Random House.

Franklin, M. E. & Foa, E. B. (2011). Treatment of obsessive compulsive disorder. *Annual Review of Clinical Psychology, 7*, 229–243.

Frost, R. O., & Steketee, G. (Eds.). (2002). *Cognitive approaches to obsessions and compulsions: Theory, assessment, and treatment.* Oxford, UK: Elsevier.

Goodman, W. K., Price, L. H., Rasmussen, S. A., Mazure, C., Fleischmann, R. L., Hill, C. L., et al. (1989). The Yale–Brown Obsessive Compulsive Scale: I. Development, use, and reliability. *Archives of General Psychiatry, 46*(11), 1006–1011.

Grados, M. A. (2003). Obsessive-compulsive disorder after traumatic brain injury. *International Review of Psychiatry, 15*(4), 350–358.

Hayes, S. C., Strosahl, K. D., & Wilson, K. G. (2012). *Acceptance and commitment therapy: An experiential approach to behavior change (2nd ed.): The process and practice of mindful change.* New York: Guilford Press.

Husted, D. S., & Shapira, N. A. (2004). A review of the treatment for refractory obsessive–compulsive disorder: From medicine to deep brain stimulation. *CNS Spectrums, 9*(11), 833–847.

Kader, M. A., Esmaeel, M. K., Nagy, N. E., & Hatata, H. A. (2013). Neurological soft signs and cognitive impairment in obsessive–compulsive disorder patients and their first-degree relatives. *Middle East Current Psychiatry, 20*(1), 35–41.

Kelley, M. L., Noell, G., & Reitman, D. (Eds.). (2003). *Practitioner's guide to empirically based measures of school behavior*. New York: Kluwer Academic/Plenum Publishers.

Kessler, R. C., Berglund, P., Demler, O., Jin, R., Merikangas, K. R., & Walters, E. E. (2005). Lifetime prevalence and age-of-onset distributions of DSM-IV disorders in the National Comorbidity Survey Replication. *Archives of General Psychiatry, 62*, 593–602.

Kim, C. H., Koo, M. S., Cheon, K. A., Ryu, Y. H., Lee, J. D., & Lee, H. S. (2003). Dopamine transporter density of basal ganglia assessed with [$^{123}$I] IPT SPET in obsessive–compulsive disorder. *European Journal of Nuclear Medicine and Molecular Imaging, 30*(12), 1637–1643.

Kircanski, K., Mortazavi, A., Castriotta, N., Baker, A. S., Mystkowski, J. L., Yi, R., et al. (2012). Challenges to the traditional exposure paradigm: Variability in exposure therapy for contamination fears. *Journal of Behavior Therapy and Experimental Psychiatry, 43*(2), 745–751.

Klinger, E. (1978). Modes of normal conscious flow. In K. S. Pope & J. L. Singer (Eds.), *The stream of consciousness* (pp. 225–258). New York: Plenum Press.

Klinger, E. (1996). The contents of thoughts: Interference as the downside of adaptive normal mechanisms in thought flow. In I. G. Sarason, G. R. Pierce, & B. R. Sarason (Eds.), *Cognitive interference: Theories, methods, and findings* (pp. 3–23). Mahwah, NJ: Erlbaum.

Koran, L. M., Theinemann, M., & Davenport, R. (1996). Quality of life in patients with obsessive compulsive disorder. *American Journal of Psychiatry, 156*, 783–788.

Kushner, M. G., Kim, S. W., Donahue, C., Thuras, P., Adson, D., Kotlyar, M., et al. (2007). D-Cycloserine augmented exposure therapy for obsessive–compulsive disorder. *Biological Psychiatry, 62*(8), 835–838.

Lazarus, A. A., & Lazarus, C. N. (1991). *Multimodal life history inventory*. Champaign, IL: Research Press.

Ledley, D. R., Marx, B. P., & Heimberg, R. G. (2010). *Making cognitive-behavioral therapy work: Clinical process for new practitioners* (2nd ed.). New York: Guilford Press.

March, J. S., Frances, A., Carpenter, D., & Kahn, D. A. (1997). The Expert Consensus Guidelines Series: Treatment of obsessive–compulsive disorder. *Journal of Clinical Psychiatry, 58*(Suppl. 4), 1–72.

Mataix-Cols, D., Frost, R. O., Pertusa, A., Clark, L. A., Saxena, S., Leckman, J. F., et al. (2010). Hoarding disorder: A new diagnosis for DSM-V? *Depression and Anxiety, 27*(6), 556–572.

McLean, P. D., Whittal, M. L., Thordarson, D. S., Taylor, S., Söchting, I., Koch, W. J., et al. (2001). Cognitive versus behavior therapy in the group treatment of obsessive–compulsive disorder. *Journal of Consulting and Clinical Psychology, 69*(2), 205–214.

Miller, W. R., & Rollnick, S. (2002). *Motivational interviewing: Preparing people for change*. New York: Guilford Press.

Nangle, D. W., Hansen, D. J., Erdley, C. A., & Norton, P. J. (2010). *Practitioner's guide to empirically based measures of social skills*. New York: Springer.

Nathan, P. E., & Gorman, J. M. (Eds.). (2015). *A guide to treatments that work* (4th ed.). New York: Oxford University Press.

National Institute for Health and Clinical Excellence (2005). Obsessive–compulsive disorder: Core interventions in the treatment of obsessive–compulsive disorder and body dysmorphic disorder (NICE Clinical Guideline 31). Available at *www.nice.org.uk/guidance/cg031*.

National Institutes of Health. (2013, March 29). NIH Fact Sheets: Obsessive–compulsive disorder. *NIH Research Portfolio Online Reporting Tools (RePORT)*. Available at *http://report.nih.gov/nihfactsheets/viewfactsheet.aspx?csid=54*.

Neziroglu, F., McKay, D., Yaryura-Tobias, J. A., Stevens, K. P., & Todaro, J. (1999). The Overvalued Ideas Scale: Development, reliability and validity in obsessive–compulsive disorder. *Behaviour Research and Therapy, 37*(9), 881–902.

Nezu, A. M., Ronan, G. F., Meadows, E. A., & McClure, K. S. (Eds.). (2000). *Practitioner's guide to empirically-based measures of depression*. New York: Springer.

Otto, M. W., Smits, J. A., & Reese, H. E. (2006). Combined psychotherapy and pharmacotherapy for mood and anxiety disorders in adults: Review and analysis. *FOCUS:The Journal of Lifelong Learning in Psychiatry, 4*(2), 204–214.

Pittenger, C., Bloch, M. H., & Williams, K. (2011). Glutamate abnormalities in obsessive compulsive disorder: Neurobiology, pathophysiology, and treatment. *Pharmacology and Therapeutics, 132*(3), 314–332.

Purdon, C. (2004). Empirical investigations of thought suppression in OCD. *Journal of Behavior Therapy and Experimental Psychiatry, 35*(2), 121–136.

Purdon, C., & Clark, D. A. (2001). Suppression of obsession-like thoughts in nonclinical individuals: Impact on thought frequency, appraisal and mood state. *Behaviour Research and Therapy, 39*, 1163–1181.

Purdon, C., & Clark, D. A. (2005). *Overcoming obsessive thoughts: How to gain control of your OCD*. Oakland, CA: New Harbinger.

Radomsky, A. S., Alcolado, G. M., Abramowitz, J. S., Alonso, P., Belloch, A., Bouvard, M., et al. (2014). Part 1—You can run but you can't hide: Intrusive thoughts on six continents. *Journal of Obsessive–Compulsive and Related Disorders, 3*(3), 269–279.

Rees, C. S., & Anderson, R. A. (2013). A review of metacognition in psychological models of obsessive–compulsive disorder. *Clinical Psychologist, 17*(1), 1–8.

Rosen, H. (1989). Piagetian theory and cognitive therapy. In A. Freeman, K. M. Simon, L. E. Beutler, & H. Arkowitz (Eds.), *Comprehensive handbook of cognitive therapy* (pp. 189–212). New York: Plenum Press.

Rosso, G., Albert, U., Asinari, G. F., Bogetto, F., & Maina, G. (2012). Stressful life events and obsessive–compulsive disorder: Clinical features and symptom dimensions. *Psychiatry Research, 197*(3), 259–264.

Saxena, S., & Rauch, S. L. (2000). Functional neuroimaging and the neuroanatomy of obsessive–compulsive disorder. *Psychiatric Clinics of North America, 23*(3), 563–586.

Simpson, H. B., Liebowitz, M. R., Foa, E. B., Kozak, M. J., Schmidt, A. B., Rowan, V., et al. (2004). Post-treatment effects of exposure therapy and clomipramine in obsessive–compulsive disorder. *Depression and Anxiety, 19*(4), 225–233.

Sookman, D., & Pinard, G. (1999). Integrative cognitive therapy for obsessive compulsive disorder: A focus on multiple schemas. *Cognitive and Behavioral Practice, 6*, 351–361.

Sookman, D., & Pinard, G. (2002). Overestimation of threat and intolerance of uncertainty in obsessive compulsive disorder. In R. O. Frost & G. Steketee (Eds.), *Cognitive approaches to obsessions and compulsions: Theory, assessment and treatment* (pp. 63–89). Oxford, UK: Elsevier.

Sookman, D., & Pinard, G. (2007). Specialized cognitive behavior therapy for resistant obsessive–compulsive disorder: Elaboration of a schema-based model. In L. P. Riso, P. L. du Toit, D. J. Stein, & J. E. Young (Eds.), *Cognitive schemas and core beliefs in psychological problems: A scientist-practitioner guide* (pp. 93–109). Washington, DC: American Psychological Association.

Sookman, D., Pinard, G., & Beauchemin, N. (1994). Multidimensional schematic restructuring treatment for obsessions. Theory and practice. *Journal of Cognitive Psychotherapy, 8*, 175–194.

Sookman, D., & Steketee, G. (2007). Directions in specialized cognitive behavior therapy for resistant obsessive–compulsive disorder: Theory and practice of two approaches. *Cognitive and Behavioral Practice, 14*(1), 1–17.

Steketee, G., & Frost, R. O. (1994). Measurement of risk-taking in obsessive–compulsive disorder. *Behavioural and Cognitive Psychotherapy, 22*(4), 287–298.

Stewart, S. E., Yu, D., Scharf, J. M., Neale, B. M., Fagerness, J. A., Mathews, C. A., et al. (2013). Genome-wide association study of obsessive–compulsive disorder. *Molecular Psychiatry, 18*(7), 788–798.

Twohig, M. P. (2004). ACT for OCD: Abbreviated treatment manual. Available at *http://contextualscience.org/files/ACT_OCD.doc*.

Twohig, M. P. (2009). The application of acceptance and commitment therapy to obsessive–compulsive disorder. *Cognitive and Behavioral Practice, 16*(1), 18–28.

Twohig, M. P., Hayes, S. C., & Masuda, A. (2006). Increasing willingness to experience obsessions: Acceptance and commitment therapy as a treatment for obsessive–compulsive disorder. *Behavior Therapy, 37*(1), 3–13.

Twohig, M. P., Hayes, S. C., Plumb, J. C., Pruitt, L. D., Collins, A. B., Hazlett-Stevens, H., et al. (2010). A randomized clinical trial of acceptance and commitment therapy versus progressive relaxation training for obsessive–compulsive disorder. *Journal of Consulting and Clinical Psychology,78*(5), 705–716.

Van Oppen, P., & Arntz, A. (1994). Cognitive therapy for obsessive–compulsive disorder. *Behaviour Research and Therapy, 32*(1), 79–87.

van Oppen, P., de Haan, E., van Balkom, A., Spinhoven, P., Hoogduin, K., & van Dyck, R. (1995). Cognitive therapy and exposure in vivo in the treatment of obsessive compulsive disorder. *Behaviour Research and Therapy, 33,* 379–390.

Wells, A. (2000). *Emotional disorders and metacognition: Innovative cognitive therapy.* Chichester, UK: Wiley.

Wells, A. (2005). Detached mindfulness in cognitive therapy: A metacognitive analysis and ten techniques. *Journal of Rational-Emotive and Cognitive-Behavior Therapy, 23*(4), 337–355.

Wells, A. (2011). *Metacognitive therapy for anxiety and depression.* New York: Guilford Press.

Whittal, M. L., Thordarson, D. S., & McLean, P. D. (2005). Treatment of obsessive–compulsive disorder: Cognitive behavior therapy vs. exposure and response prevention. *Behaviour Research and Therapy, 43*(12), 1559–1576.

Wilhelm, S., Buhlmann, U., Tolin, D., Meunier, S., Pearlson, G., Reese, H., et al. (2008). Augmentation of behavior therapy with D-Cycloserine for obsessive–compulsive disorder. *American Journal of Psychiatry, 165*(3), 335–341.

# Index

Note: *f* following a page number indicates a figure.